I0790580

**ISBN:** 9781675142752

# 30-DAY
# GLUTEN FREE
## QUICK DIET

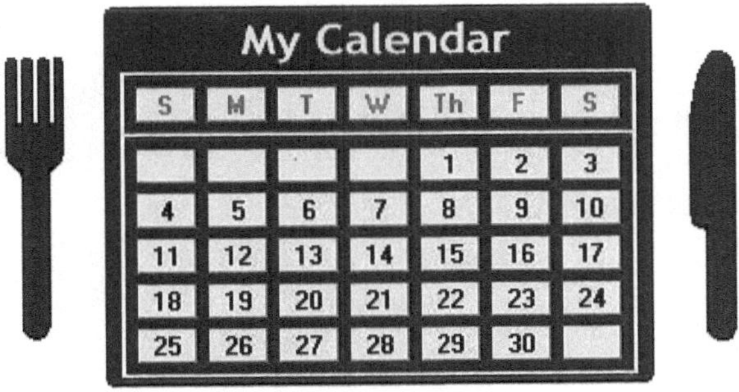


**Gail Johnson, M.S.**

**NoPaperPress™**

Note: At publication, off-the-shelf foods used in this book were widely available in most supermarkets. But food products come and go. So if there is a frozen entrée or soup selection in this diet that is out of stock, or that's been discontinued, or perhaps you don't like, or that you forgot to pick up while shopping, please substitute another food that has **approximately** the same caloric value and nutritional content. In addition, frozen entrée and soup ingredients sometimes are changed by the manufacturer without notice and without changing the product's name but the calorie count may have been increased or decreased. So make sure you check the calories noted on the food or soup container, and if the calorie value is different than shown in this book make an allowance for the calorie difference or substitute another frozen entrée or soup. In this regard, many dieters have found the many frozen foods and soups listed in the Appendices at the end of this book to be helpful.

# CONTENTS

Gluten is a mixture of two proteins that are present in wheat, barley and rye. Gluten causes harmful reactions to people who have celiac disease or are gluten sensitive. But gluten is difficult to avoid, because wheat is the third largest crop in the U.S. (behind corn and soybeans). When the acreage for wheat, barley and rye are combined, more farm acres are used to grow gluten grain crops than any other, with about 4 billion bushels of gluten grains grown in 2011. Because wheat, barley and rye grains are everywhere in our food chain, eating gluten-free involves more complicated than just substituting gluten-free bread for the usual gluten-containing bread for sale on supermarket shelves.

Another problem is gluten cross contamination which occurs when a gluten-free food comes in contact with a food that contains gluten. Cross contamination can happen at a farm where the food is grown, at a manufacturing facility where the food is processed, at a supermarket where a food may be re-packaged, and in your kitchen.

Gluten-free means that a food does not contain the gluten in wheat, barley or rye and sometimes cross-contaminated oats or soy.

## Why Gluten Free?

The primary reason for a gluten-free diet is to combat celiac disease which is a chronic, systemic, autoimmune disorder that causes intestinal damage. For more on celiac disease see **Appendix A** - page 111.

Another reason to go gluten free is to combat a condition called non-celiac gluten sensitivity that can also affect nearly every system in your body with symptoms that include digestive complaints, skin problems, brain fog, joint pain and numbness in extremities. Still another reason for a gluten-free diet is to combat a wheat allergy. For more on non-celiac gluten sensitivity see Appendix A.

A new reason to go gluten free is that many adults claim that going gluten free not only helped them lose weight but they also felt a lot better. For more on this again see Appendix A.

## Is This Diet For You?

The *30-Day Gluten-Quick Diet* is for adult men and women:
   - **With celiac disease who want to lose weight.**
   - **With gluten sensitivity or a wheat allergy who want to lose weight.**
   - **Who just want to lose weight and feel better on a gluten-free diet.**
The low-calorie menus assure that you will lose weight, while going gluten free is a healthy bonus that also makes many people feel better while on the diet.

## Choose Your Calorie Level

This eBook contains two 30-day diets: a 1,200-Calorie diet and a 1,500-Calorie diet.  And both diets have a meal plan (menu) for each and every one of the 30 days.  Which diet calorie level should you choose?

    **1,200-Calorie Diet** is **appropriate for most women**.  But due to the relatively low calorie level, you might occasionally feel hungry.  (The 1,500-Calorie diet might be a better choice for some larger, younger, or more active women.)

    **1,500-Calorie Diet** is **suitable for most men**.  This is a reasonable diet calorie level where most adults easily get all the nutrients and micro nutrients they need – and rarely feel hungry.  (The 1,200-Calorie diet might be a better choice for some smaller, or older, or inactive men.)

## Expected Weight Loss

Weight loss  occurs when your food energy intake is less than the total energy you expend. This difference in calories is referred to as your calorie deficit. How much weight you lose depends on the magnitude of your calorie deficit.  Physiologists have long known that to lose one pound requires a deficit of approximately 3,500 Calories. Therefore, if a person's total calorie deficit over time is known, their weight loss over time can be calculated.

    On the *30-Day Gluten-Free Quick Diet*, **most women lose 10 to 15 pounds.** Smaller women, older women and less active women lose a bit less and larger women, younger women and more active women often lose more.

    On the *30-Day Gluten-Free Quick Diet*, **most men lose 15 to 20 pounds.** Smaller men, older men and less active men will lose a tad less and larger men, younger men and more active men much more.

    If you want to lose even more weight take a brisk one-hour walk every day.  This applies to both men and women.

    Exactly how much weight you will lose depends on how much you weigh, your age and your activity level.  For the full story see *Weight Control - U.S. Edition* by Vincent W. Antonetti, Ph.D.

## How to Use This eBook

**1)**  Read material in **Appendix A -** page 111.  Gluten Notes and **Appendix B** on page 114 on Gluten-Free Foods.

**2)**  Choose the calorie level that's right for you, either 1200 or 1500 Calories per day - depending on your gender, your size, your age and how active you are.

**3)**  Then to start the diet go to either:

    **Day 1 of the 1200-Calorie Diet** on page 16.

    **Day 1 of the 1500-Calorie Diet** on page 47.

## First a Medical Exam

Even though this diet adheres to the United States Department of Agriculture balanced diet recommendations, it may not be appropriate for everyone, such as individuals with illnesses such as heart disease, diabetes, etc. Make sure you check with your physician before starting this diet, or any diet. **Everyone should at the very least have a medical assessment, or exam, before starting a weight loss diet.** Why? You need to make sure your health will allow you to lower your caloric intake and increase your physical activity. Depending on your age and state of health, the medical checkup may be as simple as a visit to a physician who is familiar with your medical history, or it may be a thorough physical exam.

The physician conducting the medical exam should be made aware of and should approve the specific weight loss diet you're planning. Additionally, if you are going to engage in some sort of physical activity in conjunction with this diet and especially if you have been totally inactive, or if you have or suspect you have cardiovascular disease or other health problems, or if you are obese, or if you are 40 or older, before embarking on the physical fitness portion of your weight control program you should have a stress test supervised by a physician. Finally, your physician can tell you how much and what type of exercise is right for you, how much you should weigh, and prescribe a realistic weight- loss goal.

## Eat Smart – Gluten Free

First, please read Appendix B (page 114) "Gluten-Free Foods" which is a listing of many of the gluten-free foods that are available in supermarkets and online.

Then understand that no single food can supply all the nutrients you need in the amounts you need. Gluten free aside for the moment, the most important factors in nutrition are variety, variety, variety! **Variety is the key to a nutritious diet.** As a means of setting strategies for food selection, the U.S. Department of Health and Human Services and the Department of Agriculture issue Dietary Guidelines every five years. The latest Dietary Guidelines describe a healthy diet as one that:
- Emphasizes fruits, vegetables, whole grains, and fat-free or low-fat milk products.
- Includes fish, poultry, lean meats, beans and nuts.
- Is low in saturated fats, trans fats, cholesterol, salt (sodium) and added sugars.

The latest guidelines encourage adults to consume a variety of nutrient-dense foods and beverages within their caloric needs. The afore mentioned U.S. government agencies recommend how much should be eaten from each of the basic food groups. For detailed information on gluten-free eating see **Appendix B**.

Even though most adults can get all the vitamins and minerals they need by merely consuming a variety of nutritious foods (from the fruit group, the vegetable group, the grains group, the meat and beans group, the milk group, and the oils group), many physicians recommend a daily multi-vitamin/mineral supplement – just in case you don't eat the way you should.

Be aware that some micronutrients, such as the fat-soluble vitamin A, can be harmful if taken in large quantities. To be safe your multi-vitamin/mineral supplement should contain no more than 100 percent of the recommended dietary allowance (RDA) for each vitamin or mineral. Generally, you don't need the high doses in multi-vitamin/mineral supplements labeled "therapeutic" or "extra-strength." There may be medical reasons for taking larger amounts of a vitamin or mineral than the RDA provides, but check with your doctor first.

## Tossed Salad

One of the dinner mainstays in the *30-Day Gluten-Free Quick Diet* is a gluten-free "Tossed Salad." To prepare your "Tossed Salad" start with a bowl that has a volume of <u>at least</u> 16 ounces, or 2 cups. First add about 1 cup of either green-leaf lettuce, Romaine lettuce or a Mesclun mix. Then add at least a half cup of other veggies such as broccoli, celery, cucumber, spinach, or watercress. This vegetable combination will, on average, total about 35 Calories.

You'll be eating a "Tossed Salad" just about every day at dinnertime. Remember that variety is the key to a nutritious diet. So be sure to vary the ingredients of the salad. Top your "Tossed Salad" with <u>1½ tablespoons of a gluten-free lite salad dressing</u> that contains no more than 25 Calories per tablespoon. Some of our favorite gluten-free light salad dressings are:
   - **Annie's Lite Raspberry Vinaigrette**
   - **Ken's Lite Options Italian w/ Romano & Red Pepper**
   - **Newman's Own Lite Red Wine Vinaigrette & Olive Oil**
   - **San-J's Tamari Sesame Salad Dressing**

For more gluten-free salad dressing options see page 120. Your "Tossed Salad" with gluten-free salad dressing will cost you roughly 70 Calories but will be packed with lots of health-giving vitamins, minerals and fiber.

## About Bread

First appreciate that bread, more specifically whole-grain breads, are good sources of complex carbohydrates and dietary fiber, as well as the B vitamins thiamin, riboflavin, niacin, and folate), vitamin E, and minerals (iron, magnesium and selenium).  The gluten in wheat, barley and rye consists of two proteins that combine during baking to develop a substance that provides bread with elasticity and structure.  Gluten also helps bread dough rise into a light loaf.  Other grains do not have these characteristics, which is why it is difficult to find good gluten-free bread.

The *30-Day Gluten-Free Quick Diet* requires bread at about 70 Calories per slice.  These days many supermarkets stock gluten-free bread.  The difficult part is finding a good tasting gluten-free bread with about 70 Calories per slice.  The gluten-free bread at your local supermarket vary in taste and texture, so try different brands before deciding.  As of this writing, our favorite gluten-free bread is Udi's, particularly Udi's Whole-Grain Bread at about 65 Calories per slice.

## Substituting Foods

If there is a food listed in the *30-Day Gluten-Free Quick Diet* that you don't like, or perhaps that you forgot to pick up while shopping, you probably can exchange or substitute another food in its place – a technique used by dieticians.  Exchanging a food listed in a diet for another food with approximately equal caloric value and nutritional content is the foundation of many successful long-term diets.  Substitution possibilities are almost endless but have to be done carefully.  The easiest substitutions are those within the same food group, such as exchanging one vegetable variety for another, or a glass of milk for a cup of yogurt.  More sophisticated exchanges cross food groups, such as replacing 3½ ounces of turkey with a tablespoon of peanut butter on a piece of whole-wheat bread. Both foods are complete protein and both contain about 175 Calories.  With some understanding and experience, you can substitute foods called for in this diet with equal calorie foods from the same food group.

**Breakfast**: You may substitute any cereal for any other gluten-free cereal.  For example, if you're not crazy about having Kellogg's Rice Krispies - gluten-free for breakfast on Day 4, substitute General Mills Corn Chex, etc.  But remember to adjust the amount of cereal to account for the calorie difference between brands.  (See page 115 for a list of gluten-free cereals.)  And if you don't like the soft-boiled egg called for on Day 9, cook a fried egg instead.  And if Cantaloupe is on the menu but is not in season, replace cantaloupe with a half cup of orange juice – both contain about 50 Calories.

**Snacks**: Again, where 6 ounces of yogurt is specified you may substitute an 8-ounce glass of skim milk, but to maintain a nutritionally balanced diet keep this snack a dairy selection.  Similarly, when fruit is on the menu, you may select any type of fruit but do not stray from the fruit group.  Nuts and popcorn can be interchanged at will.  Specified convenient brand-name snacks, such as Skinny Cow ice cream bars and Orville Redenbacher's Smart Pop Popcorn should be widely available but other equivalent brands may be substituted if need be.  Just make sure the substitute snack has the same calorie count, or very close, to the specified snack.

## Two Nights – No Cooking

Everyone deserves a break from the grind of preparing dinner after coming home from work.  So the *30-Day Gluten-Free Quick Diet* gives you two days off almost every week!  One night a week the meal plan calls for a frozen dinner and on a second night you are encouraged to eat out.  There are, however, some rules and caveats involved – these are covered in the next two sections.

## Frozen Dinner Rules

In general, a frozen dinner should not be a meal in itself.  Make sure you add a salad, fruit, gluten-free bread etc.  The frozen dinner you choose should come with at least one cup of cooked vegetables.  If your frozen dinner doesn't measure up, add your own frozen, fresh or canned vegetables.  And look for dinners with no more than 800 mg of sodium.  Some reasonably good gluten-free frozen dinner choices are:

- Amy's Thai Stir-Fry (310 Calories, 420 mg sodium)
- Amy's Asian Noodle Stir Fry (300 Calories, 630 mg sodium)
- Artisan Bistro Wild Alaskan Salmon (200 Calories, 135 mg sodium)
- Artisan Bistro Savory Turkey (330 Calories, 450 mg sodium)
- Smart Ones Lemon Herb Chicken Piccata (250 Calories, 540 mg sodium)
- Smart Ones Santa Fe Style Rice & Beans (290 Calories, 660 mg sodium)
For more frozen dinner choices see page 117.

And on the days when a frozen dinner is specified, you will also be given a calorie goal for the frozen dinner.  For example, Day 5 calls for frozen dinner with a maximum allowable 340 Calories.  If you choose a frozen dinner that contains less than 340 Calories, you may spend the unused calories any way you wish.

Moreover, on those nights when you just don't have the energy or time to cook, you can always substitute a frozen dinner for the "Recipe of the Day" or the entree listed in the meal plan.  Again the substitute food should be close in calorie value to the food it replaces.

## Eating Out Challenges

You may eat out once a week.  When you're on a gluten-free reducing diet, however, eating in a restaurant can be a double challenge.  First, most restaurant portions are huge, easily totaling more than 1,000 Calories, and then many restaurants do not offer gluten-free menu selections.  On the *30-Day Gluten-Free Quick Diet*, a dinner type (i.e., fish, chicken, etc) and a calorie target are specified.  For example Day 7 of the 1,200 Calorie diet calls for a chicken dinner and allows you 530 Calories.  Follow these tips to make sure your dinning experience is both low calorie, gluten-free and pleasant.

Make sure you choose a restaurant where gluten-free food is available and where you have a fighting chance to achieve your calorie goal.  Before you go read the menu online and reduce your food choices so you can have more focused questions for the staff.  You are more likely to get a safe meal if you call the restaurant before you go to let them know of your gluten-free needs.  And call during a slow time so you can have the host's complete attention.

In the restaurant, to ensure you are served a gluten-free meal, it is important to communicate your need to eat 100 percent gluten-free assertively but amiably. Try to speak directly to the chef or manager.  Otherwise, ask your server what is in the food and how it's prepared.  Menu descriptions don't always list every ingredient.  Try to get a list of ingredients for sauces and dressings.  Inquire how gluten-free grains such as rice and risottos are cooked.  Sometimes they are cooked in broth which may contain gluten.  Confirm that separate, clean utensils and equipment will be used to prepare your meal.

Order something simple, such as broiled fish with steamed vegetables and brown rice.  Tell the waiter you want no sauce, no gravy, nothing added.  Then, knowing your calorie objective, and that most fish and chicken are about 50 Calories per ounce, most steamed vegetable servings average approximately 50 Calories per cup, and rice is about 100 Calories per ½ cup, decide how much to eat – and take the remainder home.  And consider bringing your own gluten-free salad dressing to the restaurant.   If fresh fruit is not an option, pass on dessert and have the evening snack specified in the *30-Day Gluten-Free Quick Diet* meal plan for that day.

**Eating Chinese** can be especially difficult.  Try bringing a restaurant card to the Chinese restaurant.  The cards are available online and are designed to help explain a gluten-free diet to a waiter who might not speak English.  Rice noodles prepared with vegetables or chicken are generally a safe choice.  If you have celiac disease or non-celiac gluten sensitivity, avoid brown sauce which may have a cross-contaminated soy sauce base.  Instead, ask for the dish to be prepared with a white sauce using corn starch.  And although it is customary to share dishes at a Chinese restaurant, do not permit your dinner companions to contaminate your food.  Make sure your friends do not use their gluten-contaminated spoons to serve food from your gluten-free dish.

    **Social Gatherings** can be tricky.  At a dinner party, intermingling utensils and serving dishes create a perfect environment for gluten cross contamination, that is for gluten to get in your food.  But this does not necessarily mean you should to skip the party.  Try to let your host know ahead of time about your gluten-free needs.  Do this before your host starts planning the menu.  Even better, offer to bring a few dishes to share.  This ensures that there will be at least a couple of items you can eat safely and takes a burden off of your host.  Finally, ask the host if you can serve yourself first, before serving plates become gluten contaminated.

## Important Notes

**1)**  If desired, skim milk and a sugar substitute may be added to coffee or tea. And soy or almond milk may be used instead of cow's milk.

**2)**  Fried eggs and scrambled eggs should be cooked in a pan coated with a non-stick cooking spray.  DO NOT USE butter or oil.

**3)**  On bread, corn-on-the-cob, or a baked potato, if desired, you may use a zero-calorie butter substitute spray.  (I Can't Believe It's Not Butter spray is gluten free.) DO NOT USE butter or sour cream.

**4)**  Cereals should be selected from the following gluten-free varieties: General Mills Rice Chex, General Mills Corn Chex, General Mills Vanilla Chex, General Mills Cinnamon Chex, General Mills Chocolate Chex, General Mills Apple Cinnamon Chex, General Mills Honey Nut Chex, Glutino Honey Nut, Glutino Apple Cinnamon, Kellogg's Rice Krispies - gluten-free, Bob's Red Mill Oat Meal and Gifts of Nature (Montana) Oat Meal.

**5)**  Bread:  Udi's Whole Grain Bread is a good choice and has 65 Calories per slice. These days many supermarkets stock gluten-free bread although you often can find a better selection online.  If desired, bread may be sprayed with a zero-calorie butter substitute.  DO NOT USE butter.

**6)**  Use only lean cuts of meat trimmed of all visible fat.  Poultry should be limited to chicken or turkey breasts (white meat and skinless only).

**7)**  When canned tuna or salmon is specified, use only fish packed in water.

**8)**  An unlimited amount of green salad may be eaten, but the GF salad dressing should be as specified on page 9.  (Note, in the meal plans Evoo means extra virgin olive oil.)

**9)**  Use freely as desired: clear unsweetened coffee, clear unsweetened tea, water, seltzer water, any diet soda, clear soups without fat, bouillon, and seasonings such as mustard, cinnamon, dill, herbs, red and black pepper, curry and vinegar.

**10)** On days when a leftover is specified for lunch. Eat about half as much as you ate for dinner a night or two before.

**11)** Any specified snack may be moved to any other part of the day, and/or combined with lunch or dinner.

**12)** Although it's recommended that you follow the diet days as specified, it's fine to occasionally skip a day and/or pick and choose the days you prefer. (Nutritionally, each day stands on its own.)

**13)** After you complete the 30th day on the diet, if you still want to lose more weight you may repeat the diet by starting over at Day 1.

## Keeping It Off

Within five years, more than 90 percent of all dieters regain every pound they have lost. Why? In most cases it's because after losing weight most people eventually revert to their pre-diet eating and exercising habits, and this inevitably leads to their regaining the weight they lost – and often more. Obviously after a diet you weigh less. The fact is the less you weigh, the less you need to eat to sustain your lower weight.

A study, published in the *Annals of Internal Medicine*, that followed 4,000 people for three decades suggests that in the long term, 90 percent of men and 70 percent of women will become overweight. Interestingly, half of the men and women in the study, who had made it well into adulthood without a weight problem, ultimately also became overweight and a third actually became obese. The point being that you can never become complacent. You must continually watch your weight because we are all at risk of becoming overweight.

The key to long-term weight control success is knowledge and understanding, combined of course with desire and self-discipline. Once you reach your weight goal, we suggest you read *Weight Maintenance - U.S. Edition* by Vincent Antonetti, Ph.D. (also published by NoPaperPress) – absolutely the best weight maintenance book on the market.

# 1200 Calorie Meal Plans

# Day 1 - 1200 Calorie Meal Plan

| BREAKFAST | Calories | Totals |
|---|---|---|
| Grapefruit (½) | 75 | |
| Scrambled egg | 80 | |
| Gluten-free bread (page 114) toasted (1 slice) | 70 | |
| Coffee (Notes - page 13) | 10 | 235 Cal |
| | | |
| **SNACK** | | |
| Coffee or tea | 10 | 10 Cal |
| | | |
| **LUNCH** | | |
| Ham* (2 oz) with mustard on 2 slices GF bread | 290 | |
| Pickle spear | 0 | |
| Small bunch of grapes | 65 | |
| Hot or iced tea | 10 | 365 Cal |
| * See page 118. | | |
| **SNACK** | | |
| Fresh fruit in season (apple, peach, etc) | 70 | |
| Coffee or tea | 10 | 80 Cal |
| | | |
| **DINNER** | | |
| Chicken w Peppers & Onions (Day 1 Recipe  page 78) | 250 | |
| Sautéed red peppers with onions (Day 1 recipe) | 70 | |
| Green beans - steamed | 25 | |
| Mashed cauliflower | 30 | |
| Large tossed salad w 1½ Tbsp lite GF dressing (p 122) | 70 | |
| Water with lemon wedge | 10 | 455 Cal |
| | | |
| **SNACK** | | |
| GF Ginger-Snap Cookie (page 117) | 40 | |
| Coffee or tea | 10 | 50 Cal |
| | | |
| | | 1195 Cal |

# Day 2  1200 Calorie Meal Plan

| BREAKFAST | Calories | Totals |
|---|---|---|
| Orange juice (½ cup) | 50 | |
| Rice Chex* (1 cup) + ½ cup skim milk + ½ sliced banana | 195 | |
| Coffee (See Notes - page 13) | 10 | 255 Cal |
| | | |
| * See page 115 for more GF cereals. | | |
| **SNACK** | | |
| Fresh fruit in season (apple, pear, etc) | 70 | |
| Coffee or tea | 10 | 80 Cal |
| | | |
| **LUNCH** | | |
| Soup (Appendix C - page 123) | 110 | |
| GF turkey breast* (1 oz) on 1 slice GF bread | 120 | |
| Pickle spear | 0 | |
| Lettuce & tomato slices | 20 | |
| Water | 0 | 250 Cal |
| * See page 118. | | |
| **SNACK** | | |
| Coffee or tea | 10 | 10 Cal |
| | | |
| **DINNER** | | |
| Baked Herb-Crusted Cod (Day 2 Recipe - page 79) | 230 | |
| Spinach (½ cup) steamed with garlic & drizzled with | 100 | |
| Asparagus (8 spears cooked & drained) | 25 | |
| Baked potato (medium - No Butter!) | 100 | |
| Gluten-free (GF) bread* (1 slice) | 70 | |
| Water with lemon wedge | 10 | 535 Cal |
| * See page 114. | | |
| **SNACK** | | |
| GF Cookie (page 117) | 60 | |
| Coffee or tea | 10 | 70 Cal |
| | | |
| | | 1200 Cal |

# Day 3  1200 Calorie Meal Plan

| BREAKFAST | Calories | Totals |
|---|---|---|
| Fresh or frozen strawberries (½ cup) | 25 | |
| French toast (Day 3 Recipe - page 80) | 310 | |
| GF Lite Syrup* (1 Tbsp) | 30 | |
| Coffee | 10 | 375 Cal |
| * See page 122. | | |
| **SNACK** | | |
| Coffee or tea | 10 | 10 Cal |
| | | |
| **LUNCH** | | |
| Salad (3 oz canned tuna*, 1 tsp Evoo, onions, celery) | 175 | |
| Lettuce & tomato wedges | 20 | |
| GF bread (1 slice) | 70 | |
| Fresh fruit in season (apple, peach, etc) | 70 | |
| Coffee or tea | 10 | 345 Cal |
| * See page 118. | | |
| **SNACK** | | |
| Coffee or tea | 10 | 10 Cal |
| | | |
| **DINNER** | | |
| Broiled veal chop (4 oz lean) | 200 | |
| Corn on the cob (1 medium ear) (No Butter!) | 100 | |
| Broccoli (½ cup steamed & drizzled with 1 tsp Evoo) | 70 | |
| Large tossed salad w 1½ Tbsp lite GF dressing (p 120) | 70 | |
| Water with lemon wedge | 10 | 450 Cal |
| | | |
| **SNACK** | | |
| Coffee or tea | 10 | 10 Cal |
| | | |
| | | 1200 Cal |

# Day 4  1200 Calorie Meal Plan

| BREAKFAST | Calories | Totals |
|---|---|---|
| Grapefruit (½) | 75 | |
| Rice Krispies* (1 cup) + ½ cup milk+ 1 Tbsp raisins | 200 | |
| Coffee | 10 | 285 Cal |
| | | |
| * Gluten-free variety | | |
| **SNACK** | | |
| Coffee or tea | 10 | 10 Cal |
| | | |
| **LUNCH** | | |
| GF Cottage cheese* (1 cup no fat) | 140 | |
| Tossed salad with 1½ Tbsp lite GF dressing (page 120) | 70 | |
| GF bread (1 slice) | 70 | |
| Hot or iced tea | 10 | 290 Cal |
| | | |
| * Cabot No-Fat Cottage Cheese is gluten free.  See page 119. | | |
| **SNACK** | | |
| Fresh fruit in season (peach, plum, etc) | 70 | |
| Coffee or tea | 10 | 80 Cal |
| | | |
| **DINNER** | | |
| Meat Loaf (Day 4 Recipe - page 81) | 290 | |
| One-half acorn squash (baked w ½ tsp maple syrup*) | 90 | |
| Spinach (½ cup steamed & drizzled with 1 tsp Evoo) | 70 | |
| Lettuce, tomato slices & 1 Tbsp lite GF dressing | 45 | |
| Water | 0 | 495 Cal |
| | | |
| * Pure maple syrup is naturally gluten free | | |
| **SNACK** | | |
| GF Ginger-Snap Cookie (page 117) | 40 | |
| Coffee or tea | 10 | 50 Cal |
| | | |
| | | 1210 Cal |

# Day 5  1200 Calorie Meal Plan

| BREAKFAST | Calories | Totals |
|---|---|---|
| Orange juice (½ cup) | 50 | |
| Fried egg | 80 | |
| Toasted GF raisin bread (1 slice)  page 114. | 70 | |
| Coffee | 10 | 210 Cal |
| | | |
| **SNACK** | | |
| Coffee or tea | 10 | 10 Cal |
| | | |
| **LUNCH** | | |
| Soup (Appendix C - page 123) | 150 | |
| GF bread (1 slice) | 70 | |
| Lettuce and sliced tomato with 1 Tbsp lite GF | 45 | |
| Canned pineapple (½ cup, no-sugar-added juice) | 40 | |
| Water | 0 | 305 Cal |
| | | |
| **SNACK** | | |
| GF yogurt* (6 oz, nonfat, any flavor) ( page 119) | 90 | |
| Coffee or tea | 10 | 100 Cal |
| | | |
| **DINNER** | | |
| Frozen dinner (Day 5 Recipe - page 83) | 340 | |
| Large tossed salad with 1½ Tbsp lite GF dressing | 70 | |
| GF bread (1 slice) | 70 | |
| Fresh fruit in season (apple, peach, etc) | 70 | |
| Water | 0 | 550 Cal |
| | | |
| **SNACK** | | |
| Coffee or tea | 10 | 10 Cal |
| | | |
| | | 1190 Cal |

# Day 6  1200 Calorie Meal Plan

| BREAKFAST | Calories | Totals |
|---|---|---|
| Orange juice (½ cup) | 50 | |
| Cinnamon Chex (¾ cup) + ½ cup milk + ½ banana | 215 | |
| Coffee | 10 | 275 Cal |
| | | |
| **SNACK** | | |
| Fresh fruit in season (apple, plum, etc) | 70 | |
| Coffee or tea | 10 | 80 Cal |
| | | |
| **LUNCH** | | |
| Leftover meat loaf  (½ Day 4 serving) w ketchup | 155 | |
| GF bread (1 slice) | 70 | |
| Lettuce | 10 | |
| Fresh or frozen berries (½ cup) | 50 | |
| Hot or iced tea | 10 | 295 Cal |
| | | |
| **SNACK** | | |
| Handful unsalted mixed nuts | 100 | |
| Coffee or tea | 10 | 110 Cal |
| | | |
| **DINNER** | | |
| Margherita Pizza (Day 6 Recipe - page 85) | 230 | |
| Large tossed salad with 1½ Tbsp lite GF dressing | 70 | |
| Water with lemon wedge | 10 | 310 Cal |
| | | |
| **SNACK** | | |
| Skinny Cow Chocolate Truffle Bar (ice cream) | 100 | |
| Coffee or tea | 10 | 110 Cal |
| | | |
| | | 1180 Cal |

# Day 7  1200 Calorie Meal Plan

| BREAKFAST | Calories | Totals |
|---|---|---|
| Cantaloupe (½ medium) | 50 | |
| GF Oatmeal* (½ cup) + ½ cup milk + 1 Tbsp raisins | 230 | |
| Coffee | 10 | 290 Cal |
| * See page 118. | | |
| **SNACK** | | |
| Coffee or tea | 10 | 10 Cal |
| | | |
| **LUNCH** | | |
| Soup (Appendix C - page 123) | 80 | |
| Grilled cheese sandwich (2 slices GF light cheese*) | 270 | |
| Lettuce and sliced tomato | 20 | |
| Pickle spears | 0 | |
| Water | 0 | 370 Cal |
| | | |
| * See page 119. | | |
| **SNACK** | | |
| Coffee or tea | 10 | 10 Cal |
| | | |
| **DINNER** | | |
| Eat Out – Chicken dinner (Day 7 Recipe - page 87) | | |
| Max allowable calories | 530 | 530 Cal |
| | | |
| **SNACK** | | |
| Coffee or tea | 10 | 10 Cal |
| | | |
| | | 1220 Cal |

# Day 8  1200 Calorie Meal Plan

| BREAKFAST | Calories | Totals |
|---|---|---|
| Cantaloupe (½ medium) | 50 | |
| Rice Chex (1 cup) + ½ cup skim milk + ½ banana | 195 | |
| Coffee | 10 | 255 Cal |
| | | |
| **SNACK** | | |
| Fresh fruit in season (peach, plum, etc) | 70 | |
| Coffee or tea | 10 | 80 Cal |
| | | |
| **LUNCH** | | |
| Soup (Appendix C - page 123) | 140 | |
| GF turkey breast* (1 oz) on 1 slice GF bread) | 120 | |
| Lettuce & tomato slices | 20 | |
| Hot or iced tea | 10 | 290 Cal |
| * See page 118. | | |
| **SNACK** | | |
| Coffee or tea | 10 | 10 Cal |
| | | |
| **DINNER** | | |
| Baked salmon with salsa (Day 8 Recipe - page 89) | 215 | |
| Baked summer squash and zucchini | 40 | |
| Medium tomato - sliced | 20 | |
| Brown rice* (½ cup – after cooking) | 100 | |
| Large tossed salad with 1½ Tbsp lite GF dressing | 70 | |
| Water with lemon wedge | 10 | 455 Cal |
| * See page 121. | | |
| **SNACK** | | |
| GF Popcorn - 100 Calorie Mini Bag (page 120) | 100 | |
| Coffee or tea | 10 | 110 Cal |
| | | |
| | | 1200 Cal |

# Day 9  1200 Calorie Meal Plan

| BREAKFAST | Calories | Totals |
|---|---|---|
| Orange juice (½ cup) | 50 | |
| Soft-boiled egg | 80 | |
| GF bread toasted (1 slice) | 70 | |
| Coffee | 10 | 210 Cal |
| | | |
| **SNACK** | | |
| GF yogurt (6 oz, nonfat, any flavor) | 90 | |
| Coffee or tea | 10 | 100 Cal |
| | | |
| **LUNCH** | | |
| Salad (3 oz canned tuna*, 1 tsp Evoo, onions, celery) | 175 | |
| Lettuce & tomato wedges + GF bread ( 1 slice) | 90 | |
| Coffee or tea | 10 | 275 Cal |
| * See page 118. | | |
| **SNACK** | | |
| Handful unsalted mixed nuts (page 120) | 100 | |
| Coffee or tea | 10 | 110 Cal |
| | | |
| **DINNER** | | |
| Veggie burger – (1 patty) (Day 9 Recipe - page 90) | 110 | |
| Light GF cheese slice (1 oz) | 70 | |
| GF burger bun (page 118) | 180 | |
| Beets (3 small, boiled, skinned & sliced) | 45 | |
| Fresh fruit in season (apple, peach, etc) | 70 | |
| Water | 0 | 475 Cal |
| | | |
| **SNACK** | | |
| Coffee or tea | 10 | 10 Cal |
| | | |
| | | 1180 Cal |

# Day 10  1200 Calorie Meal Plan

| BREAKFAST | Calories | Totals |
|---|---|---|
| Orange juice (½ cup) | 50 | |
| Wild blueberry pancakes (Day 10 Recipe - page 91) | 210 | |
| GF Lite Syrup* (1½ Tbsp) | 45 | |
| Coffee | 10 | 315 Cal |
| * See page 122. | | |
| **SNACK** | | |
| Coffee or tea | 10 | 10 Cal |
| | | |
| **LUNCH** | | |
| GF Peanut butter* (2 Tbsp) on 2 slices of GF bread | 330 | |
| Skim milk (4 oz) | 45 | |
| Fresh fruit in season (apple, plum, etc) | 70 | |
| Water | 0 | 445 Cal |
| * See page 120. | | |
| **SNACK** | | |
| Coffee or tea | 10 | 10 Cal |
| | | |
| **DINNER** | | |
| Broiled pork chop (about 4 oz meat - trimmed of fat) | 280 | |
| Green peas (½ cup) | 55 | |
| Tomato & cucumber salad w 1½ Tbsp GF dressing | 70 | |
| Water with lemon wedge | 10 | 415 Cal |
| | | |
| **SNACK** | | |
| Coffee or tea | 10 | 10 Cal |
| | | |
| | | 1205 Cal |

# Day 11  1200 Calorie Meal Plan

| BREAKFAST | Calories | Totals |
|---|---|---|
| Fresh sliced orange | 75 | |
| Rice Krispies* (1 cup) + ½ cup milk + 1 Tbsp raisins | 200 | |
| Coffee | 10 | 285 Cal |
| | | |
| * Gluten free variety | | |
| SNACK | | |
| Coffee or tea | 10 | 10 Cal |
| | | |
| LUNCH | | |
| GF Cottage cheese* (1 cup no fat) | 140 | |
| Large tossed salad with 1½ Tbsp lite GF dressing | 70 | |
| GF bread (1 slice) | 70 | |
| Hot or iced tea | 10 | 290 Cal |
| | | |
| * Cabot No-Fat Cottage Cheese is gluten free | | |
| SNACK | | |
| Handful unsalted mixed nuts (page 120) | 100 | |
| Coffee or tea | 10 | 110 Cal |
| * | | |
| DINNER | | |
| Grilled GF chicken sausage* (2 links 2½ oz per link) | 180 | |
| Artichoke-bean salad (Day 11 Recipe - page 90) | 190 | |
| Green beans (¼ lb – steamed) | 25 | |
| GF bread (1 slice) | 70 | |
| Water | 0 | 465 Cal |
| * See page 118. | | |
| SNACK | | |
| GF Ginger-Snap Cookie | 40 | |
| Coffee or tea | 10 | 50 Cal |
| | | |
| | | 1210 Cal |

# <u>Day 12</u>  1200 Calorie Meal Plan

| **BREAKFAST** | **Calories** | **Totals** |
|---|---|---|
| **Orange juice (½ cup)** | 50 | |
| **Scrambled egg** | 80 | |
| **GF bread toasted (1 slice)** | 70 | |
| **Coffee** | 10 | **210 Cal** |
| | | |
| **SNACK** | | |
| **GF yogurt (6 oz, nonfat, any flavor)** | 90 | **90 Cal** |
| | | |
| **LUNCH** | | |
| **Soup (Appendix C - page 123)** | 150 | |
| **Tomato slices** w ¼ cup chopped fresh basil + 1 tsp Evoo | 60 | |
| **GF bread (1 slice)** | 70 | |
| **Hot or iced tea** | 10 | **290 Cal** |
| | | |
| **SNACK** | | |
| **Coffee or tea** | 10 | **10 Cal** |
| | | |
| **DINNER** | | |
| **Eat Out – Fish dinner (Day 12 Recipe - page 91)** | | |
| **Max allowable calories** | 595 | **595 Cal** |
| | | |
| **SNACK** | | |
| **Coffee or tea** | 10 | **10 Cal** |
| | | |
| | | **1205 Cal** |

# <u>Day 13</u>  1200 Calorie Meal Plan

| BREAKFAST | Calories | Totals |
|---|---|---|
| Orange juice (½ cup) | 50 | |
| Cinnamon Chex (1 cup) + ½ cup skim milk + ½ banana | 255 | |
| Coffee | 10 | 315 Cal |
| | | |
| **SNACK** | | |
| Handful unsalted mixed nuts | 100 | |
| Coffee or tea | 10 | 110 Cal |
| | | |
| **LUNCH** | | |
| GF Turkey Hot Dog* with mustard & relish | 100 | |
| GF Hot-dog bun** | 150 | |
| Diet soda or water | 0 | 250 Cal |
| * See page 118.   ** See page 114. | | |
| **SNACK** | | |
| Coffee or tea | 10 | 10 Cal |
| | | |
| **DINNER** | | |
| Pasta w Marinara sauce (Day 13 Recipe - page 92) | 225 | |
| Large tossed salad with 1½ Tbsp lite GF dressing | 70 | |
| Fresh fruit in season (peach, plum, etc) | 70 | |
| GF bread (1 slice) | 70 | |
| Water with lemon wedge | 10 | 445 Cal |
| | | |
| **SNACK** | | |
| GF Cookie* | 60 | |
| Coffee or tea | 10 | 70 Cal |
| | | |
| * See page 117. | | 1200 Cal |

# Day 14  1200 Calorie Meal Plan

| BREAKFAST | Calories | Totals |
|---|---|---|
| Cantaloupe (½ medium) | 50 | |
| Low-Cal Smoothie  (Day 14 Recipe - page 93) | 220 | |
| Coffee | 10 | 280 Cal |
| | | |
| **SNACK** | | |
| Fresh fruit in season (apple, peach, etc) | 70 | |
| Coffee or tea | 10 | 80 Cal |
| | | |
| **LUNCH** | | |
| Grilled cheese sandwich (2 slices GF light cheese*) | 270 | |
| Pickle spear | 0 | |
| Hot or iced tea | 10 | 280 Cal |
| | | |
| * See page 123. | | |
| **SNACK** | | |
| GF Popcorn - 100 Calorie Mini Bag * page 120 | 100 | |
| Coffee or tea | 10 | 110 Cal |
| | | |
| **DINNER** | | |
| Frozen dinner (Day 5 Recipe - page 82) | 300 | |
| Large tossed salad with 1½ Tbsp lite GF dressing | 70 | |
| Water with lemon wedge | 10 | 380 Cal |
| | | |
| **SNACK** | | |
| GF Cookie | 60 | |
| Coffee or tea | 10 | 70 Cal |
| | | |
| | | 1200 Cal |

# Day 15  1200 Calorie Meal Plan

| BREAKFAST | Calories | Totals |
|---|---|---|
| Fresh or frozen strawberries (1 cup) | 50 | |
| French toast (Day 3 Recipe - page 80) | 310 | |
| GF Lite Syrup (1 Tbsp) (page 122) | 30 | |
| Coffee | 10 | 400 Cal |
| | | |
| **SNACK** | | |
| Coffee or tea | 10 | 10 Cal |
| | | |
| **LUNCH** | | |
| Salad (3 oz canned tuna, 1 tsp Evoo, onions, celery) | 175 | |
| GF bread (1 slice) | 70 | |
| Water | 0 | 245 Cal |
| | | |
| **SNACK** | | |
| Fresh fruit in season (apple, plum, etc) | 70 | |
| Coffee or tea | 10 | 80 Cal |
| | | |
| **DINNER** | | |
| London broil (Day 15 Recipe - page 94) | 320 | |
| Brown rice (½ cup – after cooking) (page 118) | 100 | |
| Steamed broccoli (1 cup – after cooking) | 50 | |
| Water | 0 | 470 Cal |
| | | |
| **SNACK** | | |
| Coffee or tea | 10 | 10 Cal |
| | | |
| | | 1215 Cal |

# Day 16  1200 Calorie Meal Plan

| BREAKFAST | Calories | Totals |
|---|---|---|
| Orange juice (½ cup) | 50 | |
| GF Oatmeal (½ cup dry) + ½ cup milk + 1 Tbsp raisins | 230 | |
| Coffee | 10 | 290 Cal |
| | | |
| **SNACK** | | |
| Fresh fruit in season (apple, plum, etc) | 70 | |
| Coffee or tea | 10 | 80 Cal |
| | | |
| **LUNCH** | | |
| Soup (Appendix C - page 123) | 110 | |
| GF bread (1 slice) | 70 | |
| Lettuce & sliced tomato with 1 Tbsp lite GF | 45 | |
| Hot or iced tea | 10 | 235 Cal |
| | | |
| **SNACK** | | |
| Coffee or tea | 10 | 10 Cal |
| | | |
| **DINNER** | | |
| Baked red snapper (Day 16 Recipe - page 95) | 215 | |
| Wild rice mix (Day 16 Recipe) (page 118) | 160 | |
| Green beans & tomato | 75 | |
| Water with lemon wedge | 10 | 460 Cal |
| | | |
| **SNACK** | | |
| GF Popcorn - Mini Bag | 100 | |
| Coffee or tea | 10 | 110 Cal |
| | | |
| | | 1185 Cal |

# Day 17 1200 Calorie Meal Plan

| BREAKFAST | Calories | Totals |
|---|---|---|
| Cantaloupe (½ medium) | 50 | |
| Fried egg | 80 | |
| GF raisin bread - toasted (1 slice) | 75 | |
| Coffee | 10 | 215 Cal |
| | | |
| **SNACK** | | |
| GF Yogurt (6 oz, nonfat, any flavor) | 90 | |
| Coffee or tea | 10 | 100 Cal |
| | | |
| **LUNCH** | | |
| Soup (Appendix C - page 123) | 180 | |
| Lettuce & tomato sandwich* (Tbsp light mayo**) | 170 | |
| Cucumber slices and carrots and celery sticks | 15 | |
| Hot or iced tea | 10 | 375 Cal |
| | | |
| * Sandwich made with GF bread.   ** See page 114. | | |
| **SNACK** | | |
| Handful unsalted mixed nuts | 100 | |
| Coffee or tea | 10 | 110 Cal |
| | | |
| **DINNER** | | |
| Cajun chicken salad (Day 17 Recipe - page 96) | 330 | |
| GF bread (1 slice) | 70 | |
| Water | 0 | 400 Cal |
| | | |
| **SNACK** | | |
| Coffee or tea | 10 | 10 Cal |
| | | |
| | | 1210 Cal |

# <u>Day 18</u>  1200 Calorie Meal Plan

| BREAKFAST | Calories | Totals |
| --- | --- | --- |
| Grapefruit (½) | 75 | |
| Corn Chex (1 cup) + ½ cup skim milk + ½ banana | 215 | |
| Coffee | 10 | 300 Cal |
| | | |
| **SNACK** | | |
| Coffee or tea | 10 | 10 Cal |
| | | |
| **LUNCH** | | |
| GF Cottage cheese* (1 cup no fat) | 140 | |
| Large tossed salad with 1½ Tbsp lite GF dressing | 70 | |
| GF bread (1 slice) | 70 | |
| Hot or iced tea | 10 | 290 Cal |
| | | |
| * Cabot No-Fat Cottage Cheese is GF | | |
| **SNACK** | | |
| Handful unsalted mixed nuts | 100 | |
| Coffee or tea | 10 | 110 Cal |
| | | |
| **DINNER** | | |
| Grilled swordfish (Day 18 Recipe - page 97) | 250 | |
| Grilled potatoes (Day 18 Recipe) | 100 | |
| Grilled cherry tomatoes (Day 18 Recipe) | 50 | |
| Spinach (½ cup) steamed w garlic & drizzled w Evoo | 50 | |
| Water with lemon wedge | 10 | 460 Cal |
| | | |
| **SNACK** | | |
| Coffee or tea | 10 | 10 Cal |
| | | |
| | | 1180 Cal |

# <u>Day 19</u>  1200 Calorie Meal Plan

| BREAKFAST | Calories | Totals |
|---|---|---|
| Grapefruit (½) | 75 | |
| Scrambled egg | 80 | |
| GF bread toasted (1 slice) | 70 | |
| Coffee | 10 | 235 Cal |
| | | |
| **SNACK** | | |
| GF Yogurt (6 oz, nonfat, any flavor) | 90 | 90 Cal |
| | | |
| **LUNCH** | | |
| Soup (Appendix C - page 123) | 100 | |
| GF turkey breast (1 oz) on 1 slice GF bread | 120 | |
| Water | 0 | 220 Cal |
| | | |
| **SNACK** | | |
| Coffee or tea | 10 | 10 Cal |
| | | |
| **DINNER** | | |
| Eat Out – Chinese food (Day 19 Recipe - page 98) | | |
| Max allowable calories | 640 | 640 Cal |
| | | |
| **SNACK** | | |
| Coffee or tea | 10 | 10 Cal |
| | | |
| | | 1205 Cal |

# Day 20  1200 Calorie Meal Plan

| BREAKFAST | Calories | Totals |
|---|---|---|
| Orange juice (½ cup) | 50 | |
| Cream of Rice (1 packet) + ½ cup milk + 1 Tbsp raisins | 230 | |
| Coffee | 10 | 290 Cal |
| | | |
| **SNACK** | | |
| Handful unsalted mixed nuts | 100 | |
| Coffee or tea | 10 | 110 Cal |
| | | |
| **LUNCH** | | |
| Left over Chinese food from Day 19 | 250 | |
| Hot or iced tea | 10 | 260 Cal |
| | | |
| **SNACK** | | |
| Coffee or tea | 10 | 10 Cal |
| | | |
| **DINNER** | | |
| Spaghetti alla Puttanesca (Day 20 Recipe - page 99) | 345 | |
| Large tossed salad with 1½ Tbsp lite GF dressing | 70 | |
| GF bread (1 slice) | 70 | |
| Water with lemon wedge | 10 | 495 Cal |
| | | |
| **SNACK** | | |
| GF Ginger-Snap Cookie page 117 | 40 | |
| Coffee or tea | 10 | 50 Cal |
| | | |
| | | 1215 Cal |

# Day 21  1200 Calorie Meal Plan

| BREAKFAST | Calories | Totals |
|---|---|---|
| Cantaloupe (½ medium) | 50 | |
| Chocolate Chex (¾ cup) + ½ cup skim milk + ½ banana | 225 | |
| Coffee | 10 | 285 Cal |
| | | |
| **SNACK** | | |
| Coffee or tea | 10 | 10 Cal |
| | | |
| **LUNCH** | | |
| GF Turkey breast (2 oz) on 2 slices GF bread | 240 | |
| Lettuce, tomato and Tbsp light mayonnaise | 35 | |
| Pickle spear | 0 | |
| Fresh fruit in season (peach, plum, etc) | 70 | |
| Water | 0 | 345 Cal |
| | | |
| **SNACK** | | |
| GF Popcorn - Mini Bag | 100 | |
| Coffee or tea | 10 | 110 Cal |
| | | |
| **DINNER** | | |
| Frozen dinner (Day 21 Recipe - page 100) | 300 | |
| Large tossed salad with 1½ Tbsp lite GF dressing | 70 | |
| Water with lemon wedge | 10 | 380 Cal |
| | | |
| **SNACK** | | |
| GF Cookie | 60 | |
| Coffee or tea | 10 | 70 Cal |
| | | |
| | | 1200 Cal |

# <u>Day 22</u>  1200 Calorie Meal Plan

| BREAKFAST | Calories | Totals |
|---|---|---|
| Fresh or frozen strawberries (1 cup) | 25 | |
| French toast (Day 3 Recipe - page 80) | 310 | |
| GF Lite Syrup | 30 | |
| Coffee | 10 | 375 Cal |
| | | |
| **SNACK** | | |
| Coffee or tea | 10 | 10 Cal |
| | | |
| **LUNCH** | | |
| Soup (Appendix C - page 123) | 110 | |
| BLT sandwich - lettuce & tomato* | 270 | |
| Pickle spears (If you find pickles that are really GF) | 0 | |
| Hot or iced tea | 10 | 390 Cal |
| | | |
| * 2 slices GF turkey bacon & 1 Tbsp GF light mayo | | |
| **SNACK** | | |
| Coffee or tea | 10 | 10 Cal |
| | | |
| **DINNER** | | |
| Shrimp & spinach salad (Day 22 Recipe - page 102) | 310 | |
| GF bread (1 slice) | 70 | |
| Water with lemon wedge | 10 | 390 Cal |
| | | |
| **SNACK** | | |
| Coffee or tea | 10 | 10 Cal |
| | | |
| | | 1185 Cal |

# <u>Day 23</u> 1200 Calorie Meal Plan

| BREAKFAST | Calories | Totals |
|---|---|---|
| Cantaloupe (½ medium) | 50 | |
| Glutino Honey Nut* (¾ cup) + ½ cup milk + ½ banana | 215 | |
| Coffee | 10 | 275 Cal |
| | | |
| * Cereal | | |
| **SNACK** | | |
| Handful unsalted mixed nuts | 100 | |
| Coffee or tea | 10 | 110 Cal |
| | | |
| **LUNCH** | | |
| GF Ham (2 oz) w mustard on 2 slices GF bread | 290 | |
| Pickle spear | 0 | |
| Hot or iced tea | 10 | 300 Cal |
| | | |
| **SNACK** | | |
| Fresh fruit in season (apple, plum, etc) | 70 | |
| Coffee or tea | 10 | 80 Cal |
| | | |
| **DINNER** | | |
| Beans & Greens Salad (Day 23 Recipe - page 103) | 260 | |
| GF bread (1 slice) | 70 | |
| Baked potato (medium) - No butter! | 100 | |
| Water | 0 | 430 Cal |
| | | |
| **SNACK** | | |
| Coffee or tea | 10 | 10 Cal |
| | | |
| | | 1205 Cal |

# Day 24  1200 Calorie Meal Plan

| BREAKFAST | Calories | Totals |
|---|---|---|
| Fresh orange sliced | 75 | |
| Soft-boiled egg | 80 | |
| GF bread -toasted (1 slice) | 70 | |
| Coffee | 10 | 235 Cal |
| | | |
| **SNACK** | | |
| GF Yogurt (6 oz, nonfat, any flavor) | 90 | |
| Coffee or tea | 10 | 100 Cal |
| | | |
| **LUNCH** | | |
| Salad – 3 oz canned salmon, 1 tsp Evoo, onions & celery | 200 | |
| Lettuce & tomato wedges | 20 | |
| GF bread ( 1 slice) | 70 | |
| Coffee or tea | 10 | 300 Cal |
| | | |
| **SNACK** | | |
| Fresh fruit in season (peach, plum, etc) | 70 | |
| Coffee or tea | 10 | 80 Cal |
| | | |
| **DINNER** | | |
| Chicken breast (5 oz - broiled) | 250 | |
| Four bean salad (½ cup) (Day 24 Recipe page 104) | 135 | |
| Large tossed salad with 1½ Tbsp lite GF dressing | 70 | |
| Water with lemon wedge | 10 | 465 Cal |
| | | |
| **SNACK** | | |
| Coffee or tea | 10 | 10 Cal |
| | | |
| | | 1190 Cal |

# Day 25 1200 Calorie Meal Plan

| BREAKFAST | Calories | Totals |
|---|---|---|
| Orange juice (½ cup) | 50 | |
| Corn Chex (1 cup) + ½ cup milk + 1 Tbsp raisins | 200 | |
| Coffee | 10 | 260 Cal |
| | | |
| **SNACK** | | |
| Coffee or tea | 10 | 10 Cal |
| | | |
| **LUNCH** | | |
| GF Cottage Cheese (1 cup no fat) | 140 | |
| Large tossed salad with 1½ Tbsp lite GF dressing | 70 | |
| GF bread (1 slice) | 70 | |
| Hot or iced tea | 10 | 290 Cal |
| | | |
| **SNACK** | | |
| Coffee or tea | 10 | 10 Cal |
| | | |
| **DINNER** | | |
| Hanger steak  (Day 25 Recipe - page 105) | 320 | |
| Roasted potatoes (Day 25 Recipe) | 120 | |
| Cherry tomatoes (Day 25 Recipe) | 20 | |
| Steamed spinach (½ cup) | 25 | |
| GF bread (1 slice) | 70 | |
| Hot or iced tea | 10 | 565 Cal |
| | | |
| **SNACK** | | |
| GF Cookie (page 117) | 60 | |
| Coffee or tea | 10 | 70 Cal |
| | | |
| | | 1205 Cal |

# Day 26 1200 Calorie Meal Plan

| BREAKFAST | Calories | Totals |
|---|---|---|
| Cantaloupe (½ medium) | 50 | |
| Fried eggs (2 eggs) | 160 | |
| GF bread - toasted (1 slice) | 70 | |
| Coffee | 10 | 290 Cal |
| | | |
| **SNACK** | | |
| GF Yogurt (6 oz, nonfat, any flavor) | 90 | |
| Coffee or tea | 10 | 100 Cal |
| | | |
| **LUNCH** | | |
| Soup (Appendix C - page 123) | 160 | |
| GF bread (1 slice) | 70 | |
| Lettuce & tomato slices | 20 | |
| Hot or iced tea | 10 | 260 Cal |
| | | |
| **SNACK** | | |
| Fresh fruit in season (apple, peach, etc) | 70 | |
| Coffee or tea | 10 | 80 Cal |
| | | |
| **DINNER** | | |
| Grilled scallops (Day 26 Recipe - page 106) | 210 | |
| Grilled polenta (Day 26 Recipe) | 125 | |
| Mushroom-steamed green beans-red onion | 45 | |
| Grilled asparagus | 10 | |
| Large tossed salad with 1½ Tbsp lite GF dressing | 70 | |
| Water | 0 | 460 Cal |
| | | |
| **SNACK** | | |
| Coffee or tea | 10 | 10 Cal |
| | | |
| | | 1200 Cal |

# Day 27  1200 Calorie Meal Plan

| BREAKFAST | Calories | Totals |
|---|---|---|
| **Orange juice** (½ cup) | 50 | |
| **Cream of Rice** (1 packet) + ½ cup milk + 1 Tbsp raisins | 230 | |
| Coffee | 10 | 290 Cal |
| | | |
| **SNACK** | | |
| Coffee or tea | 10 | 10 Cal |
| | | |
| **LUNCH** | | |
| Two servings (1 cup) left over Day 24 bean salad | 270 | |
| GF bread (1 slice) | 70 | |
| Lettuce & tomato slices | 20 | |
| Hot or iced tea | 10 | 370 Cal |
| | | |
| **SNACK** | | |
| Fresh fruit in season (apple, plum, etc) | 70 | |
| Coffee or tea | 10 | 80 Cal |
| | | |
| **DINNER** | | |
| Fettuccine  (Day 27 Recipe - page 107) | 290 | |
| Large tossed salad with 1½ Tbsp lite GF dressing | 70 | |
| GF bread (1 slice) | 80 | |
| Water | 0 | 440 Cal |
| | | |
| **SNACK** | | |
| Coffee or tea | 10 | 10 Cal |
| | | |
| | | 1200 Cal |

# Day 28  1200 Calorie Meal Plan

| BREAKFAST | Calories | Totals |
|---|---|---|
| Cantaloupe (½ medium) | 50 | |
| Low-Cal Smoothie  (Day 14 Recipe - page 95) | 220 | |
| Coffee | 10 | 280 Cal |
| | | |
| **SNACK** | | |
| Fresh fruit in season (peach, plum, etc) | 70 | |
| Coffee or tea | 10 | 80 Cal |
| | | |
| **LUNCH** | | |
| Roast beef (2 oz) sandwich on GF bread | 295 | |
| Lettuce | 0 | |
| Hot or iced tea | 10 | 305 Cal |
| | | |
| **SNACK** | | |
| Coffee or tea | 10 | 10 Cal |
| | | |
| **DINNER** | | |
| Frozen dinner (Day 28 Recipe - page 108) | 300 | |
| Large tossed salad with 1½ Tbsp lite GF dressing | 70 | |
| GF bread (1 slice) | 70 | |
| Skim milk (6 oz) | 65 | |
| Water with lemon wedge | 10 | 515 Cal |
| | | |
| **SNACK** | | |
| Coffee or tea | 10 | 10 Cal |
| | | |
| | | 1200 Cal |

# <u>Day 29</u> 1200 Calorie Meal Plan

| BREAKFAST | Calories | Totals |
|---|:---:|:---:|
| Orange juice (½ cup) | 50 | |
| Wild blueberry pancakes (Day 10 Recipe - page 89) | 190 | |
| GF Lite Syrup (1½ Tbsp) | 45 | |
| Coffee | 10 | 295 Cal |
| | | |
| **SNACK** | | |
| GF Yogurt (6 oz, nonfat, any flavor) | 90 | |
| Coffee or tea | 10 | 100 Cal |
| | | |
| **LUNCH** | | |
| Salad (3 oz canned tuna, 1 tsp Evoo, onions, celery) | 175 | |
| Lettuce & tomato wedges | 20 | |
| GF bread (1 slice) | 70 | |
| Fresh fruit in season (apple, pear, etc) | 70 | |
| Coffee or tea | 10 | 345 Cal |
| | | |
| **SNACK** | | |
| Coffee or tea | 10 | 10 Cal |
| | | |
| **DINNER** | | |
| Barbequed shrimp (Day 29 Recipe - page 109) | 160 | |
| Corn on the cob (medium) | 90 | |
| Steamed broccoli (1 cup – after cooking) | 50 | |
| Water | 0 | 300 Cal |
| | | |
| **SNACK** | | |
| Glutino Chocolate-Covered Pretzels (9) (page 117) | 140 | |
| Coffee or tea | 10 | 150 Cal |
| | | |
| | | 1200 Cal |

# Day 30  1200 Calorie Meal Plan

| BREAKFAST | Calories | Totals |
|---|---|---|
| Fresh orange sliced | 75 | |
| Chocolate Chex (¾ cup) + ½ cup milk + ½ banana | 225 | |
| Coffee | 10 | 310 Cal |
| | | |
| **SNACK** | | |
| Fresh fruit in season (apple, plum, etc) | 70 | |
| Coffee or tea | 10 | 80 Cal |
| | | |
| **LUNCH** | | |
| Soup (Appendix C - page 123) | 150 | |
| GF bread (1 slice) | 70 | |
| Raw zucchini slices, celery carrot sticks | 20 | |
| Water | 0 | 240 Cal |
| | | |
| **SNACK** | | |
| Coffee or tea | 10 | 10 Cal |
| | | |
| **DINNER** | | |
| Cheeseburger  (Day 30 Recipe - page 110) | 320 | |
| Lettuce  sliced tomato | 20 | |
| GF bun | 180 | |
| Steamed green beans | 25 | |
| Pickle spear | 0 | |
| Water | 0 | 545 Cal |
| | | |
| **SNACK** | | |
| Coffee or tea | 10 | 10 Cal |
| | | |
| | | 1195 Cal |

# 1500 Calorie Meal Plans

# Day 1 - 1500 Calorie Meal Plan

| BREAKFAST | Calories | Totals |
|---|---|---|
| Grapefruit (½) | 75 | |
| Scrambled egg | 80 | |
| GF Turkey bacon* (1 slice) | 35 | |
| Gluten-free bread (GF bread)** toasted (1 slice) | 70 | |
| Coffee (See page 13) | 10 | 270 Cal |
| * See page 118.   ** See Page 114. | | |
| **SNACK** | | |
| GF yogurt - page 119  (6 oz, nonfat, any flavor) | 90 | |
| Coffee or tea | 10 | 100 Cal |
| **LUNCH** | | |
| Ham* (2 oz) with mustard on 2 slices GF bread | 290 | |
| Pickle spear | 0 | |
| Small bunch of grapes | 65 | |
| Hot or iced tea | 10 | 365 Cal |
| * See page 118. | | |
| **SNACK** | | |
| Fresh fruit in season (apple, peach, etc) | 70 | |
| Coffee or tea | 10 | 80 Cal |
| **DINNER** | | |
| Chicken w Peppers & Onions (Day 1 Recipe  page 78) | 250 | |
| Sautéed red peppers with onions (Day 1 recipe) | 70 | |
| Green beans - steamed | 25 | |
| Mashed cauliflower | 30 | |
| Large tossed salad with 1½ Tbsp lite GF dressing* | 70 | |
| GF bread (1 slice) | 70 | |
| Skim milk (4 oz - ½ cup) | 45 | |
| Water with lemon wedge | 10 | 570 Cal |
| | | |
| * See page 120. | | |
| **SNACK** | | |
| GF Popcorn* - 100 Calorie Mini Bag (page 120) | 100 | |
| Coffee or tea | 10 | 110 Cal |
| | | |
| | | 1495 Cal |

# Day 2  1500 Calorie Meal Plan

| BREAKFAST | Calories | Totals |
|---|---|---|
| Orange juice (½ cup) | 50 | |
| Rice Chex* (1 cup) + ½ cup milk+ ½ banana | 195 | |
| GF bread toasted (1 slice) | 70 | |
| Coffee | 10 | 325 Cal |
| | | |
| * See page 115 for more GF cereals. | | |
| **SNACK** | | |
| Fresh fruit in season (apple, pear, etc) | 70 | |
| Coffee or tea | 10 | 80 Cal |
| | | |
| **LUNCH** | | |
| Soup (Appendix C - page 123) | 110 | |
| GF turkey breast (1 oz) on 1 slice GF bread | 120 | |
| Large tossed salad with 1½ Tbsp lite GF dressing* | 70 | |
| Water with lemon wedge | 10 | 310 Cal |
| | | |
| * See page 120. | | |
| **SNACK** | | |
| GF Popcorn Mini Bag (page 120) | 100 | |
| Coffee or tea | 10 | 110 Cal |
| | | |
| **DINNER** | | |
| Baked Herb-Crusted Cod (Day 2 Recipe - page 79) | 230 | |
| Spinach (½ cup) steamed with garlic & drizzled | 100 | |
| Asparagus (8 spears cooked & drained) | 35 | |
| Baked potato (medium - No Butter!) | 100 | |
| Gluten-free (GF) bread (1 slice) | 70 | |
| Water with lemon wedge | 10 | 545 Cal |
| | | |
| **SNACK** | | |
| Handful unsalted mixed nuts* | 100 | |
| Coffee or tea | 10 | 110 Cal |
| | | |
| * See page 120. | | 1480 Cal |

# Day 3  1500 Calorie Meal Plan

| BREAKFAST | Calories | Totals |
|---|---|---|
| Fresh or frozen strawberries (½ cup) | 25 | |
| French toast (Day 3 Recipe - page 80) | 310 | |
| GF Lite Syrup* (1 Tbsp) | 30 | |
| Coffee | 10 | 375 Cal |
| * See page 122. | | |
| **SNACK** | | |
| GF yogurt (6 oz, nonfat, any flavor) (page 119) | 90 | |
| Coffee or tea | 10 | 100 Cal |
| | | |
| **LUNCH** | | |
| Salad (3 oz canned tuna*, 1 tsp Evoo, onions, celery) | 175 | |
| Lettuce & tomato wedges | 20 | |
| GF bread (1 slice) | 70 | |
| Fresh fruit in season (apple, peach, etc) | 70 | |
| Coffee or tea | 10 | 345 Cal |
| | | |
| * See page 118. | | |
| **SNACK** | | |
| Handful unsalted mixed nuts (page 120) | 100 | |
| Coffee or tea | 10 | 110 Cal |
| | | |
| **DINNER** | | |
| Broiled veal chop (4 oz lean) | 200 | |
| Corn on the cob (1 medium ear) (No Butter!) | 100 | |
| Broccoli (½ cup steamed & drizzled with 1 tsp Evoo) | 70 | |
| Large tossed salad w 1½ Tbsp lite GF dressing (p 120) | 70 | |
| Water with lemon wedge | 10 | 450 Cal |
| | | |
| **SNACK** | | |
| Skinny Cow Chocolate Truffle Bar* (ice cream) | 100 | |
| Coffee or tea | 10 | 110 Cal |
| | | |
| * See page 119. | | 1490 Cal |

# Day 4  1500 Calorie Meal Plan

| BREAKFAST | Calories | Totals |
|---|---|---|
| Grapefruit (½) | 75 | |
| Rice Krispies* (1 cup) + ½ cup milk+ 1 Tbsp raisins | 200 | |
| GF bread toasted (1 slice) | 70 | |
| Coffee | 10 | 355 Cal |
| | | |
| * Gluten-free variety | | |
| **SNACK** | | |
| Fresh fruit in season (peach, plum, etc) | 70 | |
| Coffee or tea | 10 | 80 Cal |
| **LUNCH** | | |
| GF Cottage cheese* (1 cup no fat) | 140 | |
| Large tossed salad w 1½ Tbsp lite GF dressing (p 120) | 70 | |
| GF bread (1 slice) | 70 | |
| Hot or iced tea | 10 | 290 Cal |
| | | |
| * Cabot No-Fat Cottage Cheese is gluten free | | |
| **SNACK** | | |
| Handful unsalted mixed nuts - See page 120. | 100 | |
| Coffee or tea | 10 | 110 Cal |
| **DINNER** | | |
| Meat Loaf (Day 4 Recipe - page 81) | 290 | |
| One-half acorn squash (baked with ½ tsp maple | 90 | |
| Spinach (½ cup steamed & drizzled with 1 tsp Evoo) | 70 | |
| Romaine lettuce, tomato slices & 1 Tbsp lite GF | 45 | |
| Water | 0 | 495 Cal |
| | | |
| * Pure maple syrup is naturally gluten free. | | |
| **SNACK** | | |
| Two GF Oatmeal-Raisin Cookies (page 117) | 180 | |
| Coffee or tea | 10 | 190 Cal |
| | | |
| | | 1520 Cal |

# Day 5  1500 Calorie Meal Plan

| BREAKFAST | Calories | Totals |
|---|---|---|
| Orange juice (½ cup) | 50 | |
| Fried egg | 80 | |
| Toasted GF raisin bread (1 slice) (page 114) | 70 | |
| Coffee | 10 | 210 Cal |
| | | |
| **SNACK** | | |
| GF yogurt (6 oz, nonfat, any flavor) | 90 | |
| Coffee or tea | 10 | 100 Cal |
| | | |
| **LUNCH** | | |
| Soup (Appendix C - page 123) | 150 | |
| GF bread (1 slice) | 70 | |
| Lettuce and sliced tomato with 1 Tbsp lite GF | 45 | |
| Canned pineapple (½ cup, no-sugar-added juice) | 40 | |
| Water | 0 | 305 Cal |
| | | |
| **SNACK** | | |
| GF Popcorn - Mini Bag (See page 120) | 100 | |
| Coffee or tea | 10 | 110 Cal |
| | | |
| **DINNER** | | |
| Frozen dinner (Day 5 Recipe - page 82) | 340 | |
| Large tossed salad w 1½ Tbsp lite GF dressing (p 120) | 70 | |
| GF bread (1 slice) | 70 | |
| Fresh fruit in season (apple, peach, etc) | 70 | |
| Water with lemon wedge | 10 | 560 Cal |
| | | |
| **SNACK** | | |
| Raw Revolution Peanut Butter Chocolate Bar* | 200 | |
| Coffee or tea | 10 | 210 Cal |
| | | |
| * See page 117. | | 1495 Cal |

# Day 6  1500 Calorie Meal Plan

| BREAKFAST | Calories | Totals |
|---|---|---|
| Grapefruit (½) | 75 | |
| Cinnamon Chex (¾ cup) + ½ cup milk + ½ banana | 215 | |
| Toasted GF bread (2 slice2) | 140 | |
| Coffee | 10 | 440 Cal |
| | | |
| **SNACK** | | |
| Handful unsalted mixed nuts  (See page 120) | 100 | |
| Coffee or tea | 10 | 110 Cal |
| | | |
| **LUNCH** | | |
| Leftover meat loaf  (½ Day 4 serving size) w ketchup | 155 | |
| GF bread (1 slice) | 70 | |
| Lettuce | 10 | |
| Fresh fruit in season (apple, peach, etc) | 70 | |
| Hot or iced tea | 10 | 315 Cal |
| | | |
| **SNACK** | | |
| GF Popcorn - Mini Bag | 100 | |
| Coffee or tea | 10 | 110 Cal |
| | | |
| **DINNER** | | |
| Margherita Pizza (Day 6 Recipe - page 84) | 230 | |
| Large tossed salad w 1½ Tbsp lite GF dressing (p 120) | 70 | |
| Water with lemon wedge | 10 | 310 Cal |
| | | |
| **SNACK** | | |
| Raw Revolution Peanut Butter Chocolate Bar | 200 | |
| Coffee or tea | 10 | 210 Cal |
| | | |
| | | 1495 Cal |

# <u>Day 7</u> 1500 Calorie Meal Plan

| BREAKFAST | Calories | Totals |
|---|---|---|
| Cantaloupe (½ medium) | 50 | |
| GF Oatmeal* (½ cup) + ½ cup milk + 1 Tbsp raisins | 230 | |
| Coffee | 10 | 290 Cal |
| | | |
| * See page 115. | | |
| **SNACK** | | |
| Fresh fruit in season (apple, peach, etc) | 70 | |
| Coffee or tea | 10 | 80 Cal |
| | | |
| **LUNCH** | | |
| Soup (Appendix C - page 123) | 80 | |
| Grilled cheese sandwich (2 slices GF light cheese*) | 270 | |
| Lettuce and sliced tomato | 20 | |
| Pickle spear | 0 | |
| Water | 0 | 370 Cal |
| | | |
| * See page 119. | | |
| **SNACK** | | |
| Coffee or tea | 10 | 10 Cal |
| | | |
| **DINNER** | | |
| Eat Out – Chicken dinner (Day 7 Recipe - page 85) | | |
| Max allowable calories | 630 | |
| Water | 0 | 630 Cal |
| | | |
| **SNACK** | | |
| Skinny Cow Chocolate Truffle Bar (ice cream*) | 100 | |
| Coffee or tea | 10 | 110 Cal |
| | | |
| * See page 119. | | 1490 Cal |

# Day 8  1500 Calorie Meal Plan

| BREAKFAST | Calories | Totals |
|---|---|---|
| Cantaloupe (½ medium) | 50 | |
| Rice Chex (1 cup) + ½ cup milk + ½ banana + 15 raisins | 235 | |
| Coffee | 10 | 295 Cal |
| | | |
| * Always use skim milk | | |
| **SNACK** | | |
| Fresh fruit in season (peach, plum, etc) | 70 | |
| Coffee or tea | 10 | 80 Cal |
| | | |
| **LUNCH** | | |
| Soup (Appendix C - page 123) | 140 | |
| GF turkey breast* (1 oz) on 1 slice GF bread | 120 | |
| Lettuce & tomato slices | 20 | |
| Hot or iced tea | 10 | 290 Cal |
| | | |
| * See page 118. | | |
| **SNACK** | | |
| GF Popcorn - 100 Calorie Mini Bag | 100 | |
| Coffee or tea | 10 | 110 Cal |
| | | |
| **DINNER** | | |
| Baked salmon with salsa (Day 8 Recipe - page 87) | 215 | |
| Baked summer squash and zucchini | 40 | |
| Medium tomato - sliced | 20 | |
| Brown rice (½ cup – after cooking) (page 118) | 100 | |
| Large tossed salad w 1½ Tbsp lite GF dressing (p 124) | 70 | |
| GF bread (1 slice) | 70 | |
| Water with lemon wedge | 10 | 525 Cal |
| | | |
| **SNACK** | | |
| Raw Revolution Peanut Butter Chocolate Bar* | 200 | |
| Coffee or tea | 10 | 210 Cal |
| | | |
| * See page 117. | | 1510 Cal |

# Day 9  1500 Calorie Meal Plan

| BREAKFAST | Calories | Totals |
|---|---|---|
| Orange juice (½ cup) | 50 | |
| Soft-boiled egg | 80 | |
| GF bread toasted (2 slices) | 140 | |
| Coffee | 10 | 280 Cal |
| | | |
| **SNACK** | | |
| GF yogurt (6 oz, nonfat, any flavor) | 90 | 90 Cal |
| | | |
| **LUNCH** | | |
| Salad (3 oz canned tuna, 1 tsp Evoo, onions, celery) | 175 | |
| Large tossed salad with 1½ Tbsp lite GF dressing | 70 | |
| GF bread ( 1 slice) | 70 | |
| Coffee or tea | 10 | 325 Cal |
| | | |
| **SNACK** | | |
| Handful unsalted mixed nuts (page 120) | 100 | |
| Coffee or tea | 10 | 110 Cal |
| | | |
| **DINNER** | | |
| Veggie burger – (1 patty) (Day 9 Recipe - page 88) | 110 | |
| Light GF cheese slice (1 oz) (page 119) | 70 | |
| GF burger bun (page 114) | 180 | |
| Beets (3 small, boiled, skinned & sliced) | 45 | |
| Fresh fruit in season (apple, peach, etc) | 70 | |
| Water with lemon wedge | 10 | 485 Cal |
| | | |
| **SNACK** | | |
| Raw Revolution Peanut Butter Chocolate Bar | 200 | |
| Coffee or tea | 10 | 210 Cal |
| | | |
| | | 1510 Cal |

# Day 10  1500 Calorie Meal Plan

| BREAKFAST | Calories | Totals |
|---|---|---|
| Orange juice (½ cup) | 50 | |
| Wild blueberry pancakes (Day 10 Recipe - page 89) | 210 | |
| GF Lite Syrup* (1½ Tbsp) | 45 | |
| GF Turkey bacon** (2 slices) | 70 | |
| Coffee | 10 | 385 Cal |
| * See page 122.   ** See page 118. | | |
| **SNACK** | | |
| GF Yogurt (6 oz, nonfat, any flavor) | 90 | |
| Coffee or tea | 10 | 100 Cal |
| | | |
| **LUNCH** | | |
| GF Peanut butter* (2 Tbsp) on 2 slices of GF bread | 330 | |
| Skim milk (4 oz) | 45 | |
| Fresh fruit in season (apple, plum, etc) | 70 | |
| Water | 0 | 445 Cal |
| | | |
| * See page 120. | | |
| **SNACK** | | |
| Handful unsalted mixed nuts (page 120) | 100 | |
| Coffee or tea | 10 | 110 Cal |
| | | |
| **DINNER** | | |
| Broiled pork chop (about 4 oz meat - trimmed of fat) | 280 | |
| Green peas (½ cup) | 55 | |
| Tomato & cucumber salad w 1½ Tbsp GF dressing | 70 | |
| Water with lemon wedge | 10 | 415 Cal |
| | | |
| **SNACK** | | |
| GF Ginger-Snap Cookie* | 40 | |
| Coffee or tea | 10 | 50 Cal |
| | | |
| * See page 117. | | 1505 Cal |

# Day 11  1500 Calorie Meal Plan

| BREAKFAST | Calories | Totals |
|---|---|---|
| Fresh sliced orange | 75 | |
| Rice Krispies* (1 cup) + ½ cup milk + 1 Tbsp raisins | 200 | |
| GF bread - toasted (1 slice) | 70 | |
| Coffee | 10 | 355 Cal |
| | | |
| * Gluten free variety | | |
| **SNACK** | | |
| GF Popcorn - Mini Bag | 100 | |
| Coffee or tea | 10 | 110 Cal |
| **LUNCH** | | |
| GF Cottage cheese (1 cup no fat) (See page 119) | 140 | |
| Large tossed salad with 1½ Tbsp lite GF dressing | 70 | |
| GF bread (1 slice) | 70 | |
| Hot or iced tea | 10 | 290 Cal |
| | | |
| **SNACK** | | |
| Handful unsalted mixed nuts | 100 | |
| Coffee or tea | 10 | 110 Cal |
| | | |
| **DINNER** | | |
| Grilled GF chicken sausage* (2 links 2½ oz per link) | 180 | |
| Artichoke-bean salad (Day 11 Recipe - page 90) | 190 | |
| Green beans (¼ lb – steamed) | 25 | |
| GF bread (1 slice) | 70 | |
| Fresh fruit in season (apple, peach, plum, etc) | 70 | |
| Water with lemon wedge | 10 | 545 Cal |
| | | |
| **SNACK** | | |
| GF Cookie | 90 | |
| Coffee or tea | 10 | 100 Cal |
| | | |
| | | 1510 Cal |

# Day 12  1500 Calorie Meal Plan

| BREAKFAST | Calories | Totals |
|---|---|---|
| Orange juice (½ cup) | 50 | |
| Scrambled eggs (2) | 160 | |
| GF bread toasted (2 slices) | 140 | |
| Coffee | 10 | 360 Cal |
| | | |
| **SNACK** | | |
| GF Yogurt (6 oz, nonfat, any flavor) | 90 | |
| Coffee or tea | 10 | 100 Cal |
| | | |
| **LUNCH** | | |
| Soup (Appendix C - page 123) | 150 | |
| Tomato slices w ¼ cup chopped fresh basil + 1 tsp Evoo | 60 | |
| GF bread (1 slice) | 70 | |
| Hot or iced tea | 10 | 290 Cal |
| | | |
| **SNACK** | | |
| GF Popcorn - Mini Bag | 100 | |
| Coffee or tea | 10 | 110 Cal |
| | | |
| **DINNER** | | |
| Eat Out – Fish dinner (Day 12 Recipe - page 91) | | |
| Max allowable calories | 595 | 595 Cal |
| | | |
| **SNACK** | | |
| GF cookie | 60 | |
| Coffee or tea | 10 | 70 Cal |
| | | |
| | | 1525 Cal |

# <u>Day 13</u> 1500 Calorie Meal Plan

| BREAKFAST | Calories | Totals |
|---|---|---|
| Orange juice (½ cup) | 50 | |
| Cinnamon Chex (1 cup) + ½ cup milk + ½ banana | 255 | |
| GF bread - toasted (1 slice) | 70 | |
| Coffee | 10 | 385 Cal |
| | | |
| **SNACK** | | |
| Handful unsalted mixed nuts | 100 | |
| Coffee or tea | 10 | 110 Cal |
| | | |
| **LUNCH** | | |
| GF Turkey Hot Dog* with mustard & relish | 100 | |
| GF Hot-dog bun** | 150 | |
| Diet soda | 0 | 250 Cal |
| | | |
| * See page 118.   ** See page 114. | | |
| **SNACK** | | |
| GF Popcorn - Mini Bag | 100 | |
| Coffee or tea | 10 | 110 Cal |
| | | |
| **DINNER** | | |
| Pasta w Marinara sauce (Day 13 Recipe - page 92) | 225 | |
| Large tossed salad with 1½ Tbsp lite GF dressing | 70 | |
| Fresh fruit in season (peach, plum, etc) | 70 | |
| GF bread (1 slice) | 70 | |
| Water with lemon wedge | 10 | 445 Cal |
| | | |
| **SNACK** | | |
| Two GF Cookies (page 117) | 180 | |
| Coffee or tea | 10 | 190 Cal |
| | | |
| | | 1490 Cal |

# Day 14  1500 Calorie Meal Plan

| BREAKFAST | Calories | Totals |
|---|---|---|
| Cantaloupe (½ medium) | 50 | |
| Low-Cal Smoothie  (Day 14 Recipe - page 93) | 220 | |
| GF bread - toasted (1 slice) | 70 | |
| Coffee | 10 | 350 Cal |
| | | |
| **SNACK** | | |
| Fresh fruit in season (apple, peach, etc) | 70 | |
| Coffee or tea | 10 | 80 Cal |
| | | |
| **LUNCH** | | |
| Grilled cheese sandwich (2 slices GF light cheese*) | 270 | |
| Pickle spear | 0 | |
| Hot or iced tea | 10 | 280 Cal |
| | | |
| * See page 119. | | |
| **SNACK** | | |
| GF Popcorn - 100 Calorie Mini Bag (page 120) | 100 | |
| Coffee or tea | 10 | 110 Cal |
| | | |
| **DINNER** | | |
| Frozen dinner (Day 5 Recipe - page 82) | 300 | |
| Large tossed salad with 1½ Tbsp lite GF dressing | 70 | |
| GF bread (1 slice) | 70 | |
| Water with lemon wedge | 10 | 450 Cal |
| | | |
| **SNACK** | | |
| Raw Revolution Peanut Butter Chocolate Bar* | 200 | |
| Coffee or tea | 10 | 210 Cal |
| | | |
| * See page 117. | | 1480 Cal |

# <u>Day 15</u>  1500 Calorie Meal Plan

| BREAKFAST | Calories | Totals |
|---|---|---|
| Fresh or frozen strawberries (1 cup) | 50 | |
| French toast (Day 3 Recipe - page 80) | 310 | |
| GF Turkey bacon* (2 slices) | 70 | |
| GF Lite Syrup** (1 Tbsp) | 30 | |
| Coffee | 10 | 470 Cal |
| | | |
| * See page 118.   ** See page 122. | | |
| **SNACK** | | |
| Handful unsalted mixed nuts | 100 | |
| Coffee or tea | 10 | 110 Cal |
| | | |
| **LUNCH** | | |
| Salad (3 oz canned tuna, 1 tsp Evoo, onions, celery) | 175 | |
| GF bread (1 slice) | 70 | |
| Water with lemon wedge | 10 | 255 Cal |
| | | |
| **SNACK** | | |
| Fresh fruit in season (apple, plum, etc) | 70 | |
| Coffee or tea | 10 | 80 Cal |
| | | |
| **DINNER** | | |
| London broil (Day 15 Recipe - page 94) | 320 | |
| Brown rice (½ cup – after cooking) (page 117) | 100 | |
| Steamed broccoli (1 cup – after cooking) | 50 | |
| Large tossed salad with 1½ Tbsp lite GF dressing | 70 | |
| Water | 0 | 540 Cal |
| | | |
| **SNACK** | | |
| GF Ginger-Snap Cookie | 40 | |
| Coffee or tea | 10 | 50 Cal |
| | | |
| | | 1505 Cal |

# Day 16  1500 Calorie Meal Plan

| BREAKFAST | Calories | Totals |
|---|---|---|
| Orange juice (½ cup) | 50 | |
| GF Oatmeal (½ cup dry) + ½ cup milk + 1 Tbsp raisins | 230 | |
| GF bread - toasted (1 slice) | 70 | |
| Coffee | 10 | 360 Cal |
| | | |
| SNACK | | |
| Handful unsalted mixed nuts | 100 | |
| Coffee or tea | 10 | 110 Cal |
| | | |
| LUNCH | | |
| Soup (Appendix C - page 123) | 110 | |
| GF bread (1 slice) | 70 | |
| Large tossed salad with 1½ Tbsp lite GF dressing | 70 | |
| Hot or iced tea | 10 | 260 Cal |
| | | |
| SNACK | | |
| GF Popcorn - 100 Calorie Mini Bag | 100 | |
| Coffee or tea | 10 | 110 Cal |
| | | |
| DINNER | | |
| Baked red snapper (Day 16 Recipe - page 95) | 215 | |
| Wild rice* mix (Day 16 Recipe) (page 117) | 160 | |
| Green beans & tomato | 75 | |
| Fresh fruit in season (apple, plum, etc) | 70 | |
| Water with lemon wedge | 10 | 530 Cal |
| | | |
| SNACK | | |
| Skinny Cow Low Fat Bar (any flavor)* | 100 | |
| Coffee or tea | 10 | 110 Cal |
| | | |
| * Ice cream | | 1480 Cal |

# Day 17  1500 Calorie Meal Plan

| BREAKFAST | Calories | Totals |
|---|---|---|
| Cantaloupe (½ medium) | 50 | |
| Fried egg | 80 | |
| GF Turkey bacon (2 slices) | 70 | |
| GF raisin bread - toasted (1 slice) | 70 | |
| Coffee | 10 | 280 Cal |
| | | |
| **SNACK** | | |
| GF Yogurt (6 oz, nonfat, any flavor) | 90 | |
| Coffee or tea | 10 | 100 Cal |
| | | |
| **LUNCH** | | |
| Soup (Appendix C - page 123) | 180 | |
| Lettuce & tomato sandwich (Tbsp light mayo*) | 170 | |
| Cucumber slices and carrots and celery sticks | 15 | |
| Hot or iced tea | 10 | 375 Cal |
| | | |
| * See page 122. | | |
| **SNACK** | | |
| Handful unsalted mixed nuts | 100 | |
| Coffee or tea | 10 | 110 Cal |
| | | |
| **DINNER** | | |
| Cajun chicken salad (Day 17 Recipe - page 96) | 330 | |
| GF bread (1 slice) | 70 | |
| Water with lemon wedge | 10 | 410 Cal |
| | | |
| **SNACK** | | |
| Raw Revolution Peanut Butter Chocolate Bar | 200 | |
| Coffee or tea | 10 | 210 Cal |
| | | |
| | | 1485 Cal |

# <u>Day 18</u> 1500 Calorie Meal Plan

| BREAKFAST | Calories | Totals |
|---|---|---|
| Grapefruit (½) | 75 | |
| Corn Chex (1 cup) + ½ cup skim milk + ½ banana | 215 | |
| GF bread - toasted (1 slice) | 70 | |
| Coffee | 10 | 370 Cal |
| | | |
| **SNACK** | | |
| Handful unsalted mixed nuts | 100 | |
| Coffee or tea | 10 | 110 Cal |
| | | |
| **LUNCH** | | |
| GF Cottage cheese* (1 cup no fat) | 140 | |
| Large tossed salad with 1½ Tbsp lite GF dressing | 70 | |
| GF bread (1 slice) | 70 | |
| Hot or iced tea | 10 | 290 Cal |
| | | |
| **SNACK** | | |
| GF Popcorn - Mini Bag | 100 | |
| Coffee or tea | 10 | 110 Cal |
| | | |
| **DINNER** | | |
| Grilled swordfish (Day 18 Recipe - page 97) | 250 | |
| Grilled potatoes (Day 18 Recipe) | 100 | |
| Grilled cherry tomatoes (Day 18 Recipe) | 50 | |
| Spinach (½ cup) steamed w garlic & drizzled w Evoo | 50 | |
| Water with lemon wedge | 10 | 460 Cal |
| | | |
| **SNACK** | | |
| GF cookie (2 cookies) | 130 | |
| Coffee or tea | 10 | 140 Cal |
| | | |
| | | 1480 Cal |

# Day 19  1500 Calorie Meal Plan

| BREAKFAST | Calories | Totals |
|---|---|---|
| Grapefruit (½) | 75 | |
| Scrambled egg | 80 | |
| GF bread toasted (2 slices) | 140 | |
| Coffee | 10 | 305 Cal |
| | | |
| **SNACK** | | |
| | | |
| GF Yogurt (6 oz, nonfat, any flavor) | 90 | |
| Coffee or tea | 10 | 100 Cal |
| | | |
| **LUNCH** | | |
| | | |
| Soup (Appendix C - page 123) | 100 | |
| GF turkey breast (1 oz) on 1 slice GF bread | 120 | |
| Fresh fruit in season (apple, plum, etc) | 70 | |
| Water | 0 | 280 Cal |
| | | |
| **SNACK** | | |
| | | |
| Handful of unsalted mixed nuts | 100 | |
| Coffee or tea | 10 | 110 Cal |
| | | |
| **DINNER** | | |
| | | |
| Eat Out – Chinese food* (Day 19 Recipe - page 98) | | |
| Max allowable calories | 600 | 600 Cal |
| | | |
| * Order about 900 Cal.  Take home about 300 Cal for lunch | | |
| **SNACK** | | |
| | | |
| GF Popcorn - Mini Bag | 100 | |
| Coffee or tea | 10 | 110 Cal |
| | | |
| | | 1505 Cal |

# <u>Day 20</u>  1500 Calorie Meal Plan

| BREAKFAST | Calories | Totals |
|---|---|---|
| Grapefruit (½) | 75 | |
| Cream of Rice (1 packet) + ½ cup milk + 1 Tbsp raisins | 230 | |
| GF bread toasted (1 slice) | 70 | |
| Coffee | 10 | 385 Cal |
| | | |
| **SNACK** | | |
| Handful unsalted mixed nuts | 100 | |
| Coffee or tea | 10 | 110 Cal |
| | | |
| **LUNCH** | | |
| Left over Chinese food from Day 19 | 300 | |
| Hot or iced tea | 10 | 260 Cal |
| Fresh fruit in season (apple, plum, etc) | 70 | |
| | | |
| **SNACK** | | |
| GF Yogurt (6 oz, nonfat, any flavor) | 90 | |
| Coffee or tea | 10 | 100 Cal |
| | | |
| **DINNER** | | |
| Spaghetti alla Puttanesca (Day 20 Recipe - page 99) | 345 | |
| Large tossed salad with 1½ Tbsp lite GF dressing | 70 | |
| GF bread (1 slice) | 70 | |
| Water with lemon wedge | 10 | 495 Cal |
| | | |
| **SNACK** | | |
| GF cookie (2 cookies) (page 117) | 130 | |
| Coffee or tea | 10 | 140 Cal |
| | | |
| | | 1490 Cal |

# Day 21  1500 Calorie Meal Plan

| BREAKFAST | Calories | Totals |
|---|---|---|
| Cantaloupe (½ medium) | 50 | |
| Chocolate Chex (¾ cup) + ½ cup milk + ½ banana | 225 | |
| GF bread - toasted (1 slice) | 70 | |
| Coffee | 10 | 355 Cal |
| | | |
| **SNACK** | | |
| Fresh fruit in season (peach, plum, etc) | 70 | |
| Coffee or tea | 10 | 80 Cal |
| | | |
| **LUNCH** | | |
| GF Turkey breast (2 oz) on 2 slices GF bread | 240 | |
| Lettuce, tomato and Tbsp light mayo | 35 | |
| Pickle spear | 0 | |
| GF bread | 70 | |
| Water with lemon wedge | 10 | 355 Cal |
| | | |
| **SNACK** | | |
| GF Popcorn - Mini Bag | 100 | |
| Coffee or tea | 10 | 110 Cal |
| | | |
| **DINNER** | | |
| Frozen dinner (Day 21 Recipe - page 100) | 300 | |
| Large tossed salad with 1½ Tbsp lite GF dressing | 70 | |
| GF bread | 70 | |
| Water with lemon wedge | 10 | 450 Cal |
| | | |
| **SNACK** | | |
| GF cookie (2 cookies) | 130 | |
| Coffee or tea | 10 | 140 Cal |
| | | |
| | | 1490 Cal |

# Day 22  1500 Calorie Meal Plan

| BREAKFAST | Calories | Totals |
|---|---|---|
| Fresh or frozen strawberries (1 cup) | 25 | |
| French toast (Day 3 Recipe - page 80) | 310 | |
| GF Lite Syrup | 30 | |
| Coffee | 10 | 375 Cal |
| | | |
| **SNACK** | | |
| GF Yogurt (6 oz, nonfat, any flavor) | 90 | |
| Coffee or tea | 10 | 100 Cal |
| | | |
| **LUNCH** | | |
| Soup (Appendix C - page 123) | 110 | |
| BLT sandwich - lettuce & tomato* | 270 | |
| Fresh fruit in season (apple, peach, etc) | 70 | |
| Hot or iced tea | 10 | 460 Cal |
| | | |
| * 2 slices **GF turkey bacon** & 1 Tbsp **GF light mayo** | | |
| **SNACK** | | |
| GF Popcorn - Mini Bag | 100 | |
| Coffee or tea | 10 | 110 Cal |
| | | |
| **DINNER** | | |
| Shrimp & spinach salad (Day 22 Recipe - page 102) | 310 | |
| GF bread (1 slice) | 70 | |
| Water with lemon wedge | 10 | 390 Cal |
| | | |
| **SNACK** | | |
| GF cookie | 60 | |
| Coffee or tea | 10 | 70 Cal |
| | | |
| | | 1505 Cal |

# <u>Day 23</u>  1500 Calorie Meal Plan

| BREAKFAST | Calories | Totals |
|---|---|---|
| Cantaloupe (½ medium) | 50 | |
| Glutino Honey Nut* (¾ cup) + ½ cup milk + ½ banana | 215 | |
| GF bread - toasted (1 slice) | 70 | |
| Coffee | 10 | 355 Cal |
| | | |
| * Cereal | | |
| **SNACK** | | |
| | | |
| Handful unsalted mixed nuts | 100 | |
| Coffee or tea | 10 | 110 Cal |
| | | |
| **LUNCH** | | |
| | | |
| GF Ham (2 oz) with mustard on 2 slices GF bread | 290 | |
| Pickle spear | 0 | |
| Fresh fruit in season (apple, plum, etc) | 70 | |
| Hot or iced tea | 10 | 370 Cal |
| | | |
| **SNACK** | | |
| | | |
| GF Popcorn - Mini Bag | 100 | |
| Coffee or tea | 10 | 110 Cal |
| | | |
| **DINNER** | | |
| | | |
| Beans & Greens Salad (Day 23 Recipe - page 103) | 260 | |
| GF bread (1 slice) | 70 | |
| Baked potato (medium) - No butter! | 100 | |
| Water | 0 | 430 Cal |
| | | |
| **SNACK** | | |
| | | |
| Skinny Cow Low Fat Bar (any flavor) | 100 | |
| Coffee or tea | 10 | 110 Cal |
| | | |
| | | 1485 Cal |

# Day 24  1500 Calorie Meal Plan

| BREAKFAST | Calories | Totals |
|---|---|---|
| Fresh orange sliced | 75 | |
| Soft-boiled egg | 80 | |
| GF bread -toasted (2 slices) | 140 | |
| Coffee | 10 | 305 Cal |
| | | |
| **SNACK** | | |
| GF Yogurt (6 oz, nonfat, any flavor) | 90 | |
| Coffee or tea | 10 | 100 Cal |
| | | |
| **LUNCH** | | |
| Salad – 3 oz canned salmon, 1 tsp Evoo, onions & celery | 200 | |
| Lettuce & tomato wedges | 20 | |
| GF bread ( 1 slice) | 70 | |
| Fresh fruit in season (peach, plum, etc) | 70 | |
| Coffee or tea | 10 | 370 Cal |
| | | |
| **SNACK** | | |
| Handful unsalted mixed nuts | 100 | |
| Coffee or tea | 10 | 110 Cal |
| | | |
| **DINNER** | | |
| Chicken breast (5 oz - broiled) | 250 | |
| Four bean salad (½ cup) (Day 24 Recipe page 104) | 135 | |
| Large tossed salad with 1½ Tbsp lite GF dressing | 70 | |
| GF bread ( 1 slice) | 70 | |
| Water with lemon wedge | 10 | 535 Cal |
| | | |
| **SNACK** | | |
| GF cookie | 90 | |
| Coffee or tea | 10 | 100 Cal |
| | | |
| | | 1520 Cal |

# Day 25  1500 Calorie Meal Plan

| BREAKFAST | Calories | Totals |
|---|---|---|
| Orange juice (½ cup) | 50 | |
| Corn Chex (1 cup) + ½ cup milk + 1 Tbsp raisins | 200 | |
| GF bread - toasted (1 slice) | 70 | |
| Coffee | 10 | 330 Cal |
| | | |
| **SNACK** | | |
| Fresh fruit in season (peach, plum, etc) | 70 | |
| Coffee or tea | 10 | 80 Cal |
| | | |
| **LUNCH** | | |
| GF Cottage Cheese (1 cup no fat) | 140 | |
| Large tossed salad with 1½ Tbsp lite GF dressing | 70 | |
| GF bread (1 slice) | 70 | |
| Hot or iced tea | 10 | 290 Cal |
| | | |
| **SNACK** | | |
| GF Popcorn - Mini Bag | 100 | |
| Coffee or tea | 10 | 110 Cal |
| | | |
| **DINNER** | | |
| Hanger steak  (Day 25 Recipe - page 105) | 320 | |
| Roasted potatoes (Day 25 Recipe) | 120 | |
| Cherry tomatoes (Day 25 Recipe) | 20 | |
| Steamed spinach (½ cup) | 25 | |
| GF bread (1 slice) | 70 | |
| Hot or iced tea | 10 | 565 Cal |
| | | |
| **SNACK** | | |
| GF cookie (2 cookies) | 120 | |
| Coffee or tea | 10 | 130 Cal |
| | | |
| | | 1505 Cal |

# Day 26  1500 Calorie Meal Plan

| BREAKFAST | Calories | Totals |
|---|---|---|
| Cantaloupe (½ medium) | 50 | |
| Fried eggs (2 eggs) | 160 | |
| GF Turkey bacon (2 slices) | 70 | |
| GF bread - toasted (2 slices) | 140 | |
| Coffee | 10 | 430 Cal |
| | | |
| **SNACK** | | |
| GF Yogurt (6 oz, nonfat, any flavor) | 90 | |
| Coffee or tea | 10 | 100 Cal |
| | | |
| **LUNCH** | | |
| Soup (Appendix C - page 123) | 160 | |
| GF bread (1 slice) | 70 | |
| Fresh fruit in season (apple, peach, etc) | 70 | |
| Hot or iced tea | 10 | 310 Cal |
| | | |
| **SNACK** | | |
| Handful unsalted mixed nuts | 100 | |
| Coffee or tea | 10 | 110 Cal |
| | | |
| **DINNER** | | |
| Grilled scallops (Day 26 Recipe - page 106) | 210 | |
| Grilled polenta (Day 26 Recipe) | 125 | |
| Mushroom-steamed green beans-red onion | 45 | |
| Grilled asparagus | 10 | |
| Large tossed salad with 1½ Tbsp lite GF dressing | 70 | |
| Water | 0 | 460 Cal |
| | | |
| **SNACK** | | |
| Skinny Cow Low Fat Bar (any flavor) | 100 | |
| Coffee or tea | 10 | 110 Cal |
| | | |
| | | 1520 Cal |

# Day 27  1500 Calorie Meal Plan

| BREAKFAST | Calories | Totals |
|---|---|---|
| Orange juice (½ cup) | 50 | |
| **Cream of Rice** (1 packet) + ½ cup milk + 1 Tbsp raisins | 230 | |
| GF bread - toasted (1 slice) | 70 | |
| Coffee | 10 | 360 Cal |
| | | |
| SNACK | | |
| Coffee or tea | 10 | 10 Cal |
| | | |
| LUNCH | | |
| Two servings (1 cup) left over Day 24 bean salad | 270 | |
| GF bread (1 slice) | 70 | |
| Fresh fruit in season (pear, plum, etc) | 70 | |
| Water | 0 | 410 Cal |
| | | |
| SNACK | | |
| GF Yogurt (6 oz, nonfat, any flavor) | 90 | |
| Coffee or tea | 10 | 100 Cal |
| | | |
| DINNER | | |
| Fettuccine  (Day 27 Recipe - page 107) | 290 | |
| Large tossed salad with 1½ Tbsp lite GF dressing | 70 | |
| GF bread (1 slice) | 70 | |
| Water | 0 | 430 Cal |
| | | |
| SNACK | | |
| Raw Revolution Peanut Butter Chocolate Bar | 200 | |
| Coffee or tea | 10 | 210 Cal |
| | | |
| | | 1520 Cal |

# <u>Day 28</u>  1500 Calorie Meal Plan

| BREAKFAST | Calories | Totals |
|---|---|---|
| Cantaloupe (½ medium) | 50 | |
| Low-Cal Smoothie  (Day 14 Recipe - page 93) | 220 | |
| Coffee | 10 | 280 Cal |
| | | |
| **SNACK** | | |
| Handful unsalted mixed nuts | 100 | 100 Cal |
| | | |
| **LUNCH** | | |
| Roast beef (2 oz) sandwich on GF bread | 295 | |
| Fresh fruit in season (peach, plum, etc) | 70 | |
| Hot or iced tea | 10 | 375 Cal |
| | | |
| **SNACK** | | |
| GF Popcorn - Mini Bag | 100 | |
| Coffee or tea | 10 | 110 Cal |
| | | |
| **DINNER** | | |
| Frozen dinner (Day 28 Recipe - page 108) | 300 | |
| Large tossed salad with 1½ Tbsp lite GF dressing | 70 | |
| GF bread (1 slice) | 70 | |
| Glass wine (4 oz) | 100 | |
| Water | 0 | 540 Cal |
| | | |
| **SNACK** | | |
| GF cookie | 90 | |
| Coffee or tea | 10 | 100 Cal |
| | | |
| | | 1505 Cal |

# Day 29  1500 Calorie Meal Plan

| BREAKFAST | Calories | Totals |
|---|---|---|
| Orange juice (½ cup) | 50 | |
| Wild blueberry pancakes (Day 10 Recipe - page 91) | 190 | |
| GF Turkey bacon (2 slices) | 70 | |
| GF Lite Syrup (1½ Tbsp) | 45 | |
| Coffee | 10 | 365 Cal |
| | | |
| SNACK | | |
| GF Yogurt (6 oz, nonfat, any flavor) | 90 | |
| Coffee or tea | 10 | 100 Cal |
| | | |
| LUNCH | | |
| Salad (3 oz canned tuna, 1 tsp Evoo, onions, celery) | 175 | |
| Lettuce & tomato wedges | 20 | |
| GF bread (1 slice) | 70 | |
| Fresh fruit in season (apple, pear, etc) | 70 | |
| Hot or iced tea | 10 | 345 Cal |
| | | |
| SNACK | | |
| Handful unsalted mixed nuts | 100 | |
| Coffee or tea | 10 | 110 Cal |
| | | |
| DINNER | | |
| Barbequed shrimp (Day 29 Recipe - page 109) | 160 | |
| Large tossed salad with 1½ Tbsp lite GF dressing | 70 | |
| Corn on the cob (medium) | 90 | |
| Steamed broccoli (1 cup – after cooking) | 50 | |
| Water | 0 | 370 Cal |
| | | |
| SNACK | | |
| Raw Revolution Peanut Butter Chocolate Bar | 200 | |
| Coffee or tea | 10 | 210 Cal |
| | | |
| | | 1500 Cal |

# Day 30  1500 Calorie Meal Plan

| BREAKFAST | Calories | Totals |
|---|---|---|
| Fresh orange sliced | 75 | |
| Chocolate Chex (¾ cup) + ½ cup skim milk + ½ banana | 225 | |
| GF bread - toasted (1 slice) | 70 | |
| Coffee | 10 | 380 Cal |
| | | |
| **SNACK** | | |
| Fresh fruit in season (apple, plum, etc) | 70 | |
| Coffee or tea | 10 | 80 Cal |
| | | |
| **LUNCH** | | |
| Soup (Appendix C - page 123) | 150 | |
| GF bread (1 slice) | 70 | |
| Raw zucchini slices, celery & carrot sticks | 25 | |
| Coffee or tea | 10 | 255 Cal |
| | | |
| **SNACK** | | |
| GF Popcorn - Mini Bag | 100 | |
| Coffee or tea | 10 | 110 Cal |
| | | |
| **DINNER** | | |
| Cheeseburger  (Day 30 Recipe - page 110) | 320 | |
| Lettuce and sliced tomato | 20 | |
| GF burger bun | 180 | |
| Steamed green beans | 25 | |
| Water with lemon wedge | 10 | 555 Cal |
| | | |
| **SNACK** | | |
| Skinny Cow Low Fat Bar (any flavor) | 100 | |
| Coffee or tea | 10 | 110 Cal |
| | | |
| | | 1490 Cal |

# Recipes & Diet Tips

## <u>Day 1 - Chicken with Peppers & Onions</u>

   4 boneless and skinless chicken breasts (about 5 oz each)
Coat the chicken breasts in a bottled barbeque sauce.  Prepare medium-hot
fire on well-oiled grill.  Place breasts on grill, turning them every 4 minutes,
for 10 to 12 minutes, or until done.  (To check if breasts are done, the meat
should be moist and white with no sign of pink when you cut into the breast.)
Salt and pepper to taste.
   2  medium red peppers, sliced
   1  medium onion, sliced
Place peppers and onions in pan with 2 tablespoons fat-free **gluten-free
chicken stock** (see page 125).  Sauté until stock is reduced.  Spray pan
lightly with **non-stick cooking oil** (page 123) and cook another 2 minutes.
Salt and pepper to taste.
<u>Serves 4</u>.  About 250 Calories per serving (for chicken only).

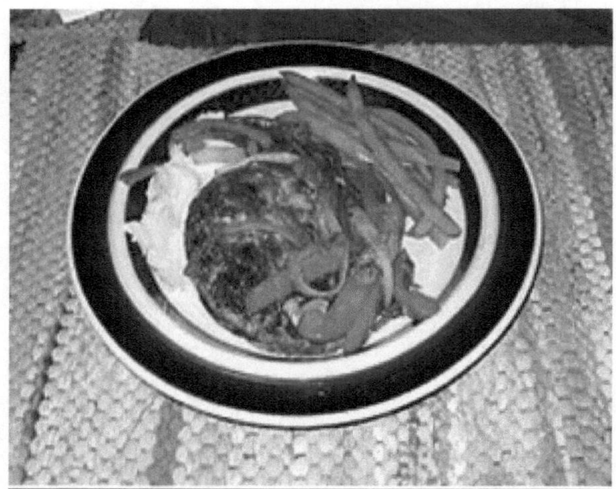

<u>Diet Tip of the Day:</u>  Weight Loss – take it one step, one meal, one workout,
one day at a time.  Just think of where you'll be in 90 days!

## <u>Day 2 - Baked Herb-Crusted Cod</u>

    4  cod fish fillets (4 to 5 ounces each)
    2  tablespoons **all-purpose GF free flour** (page 117)
    2  tablespoons GF cornmeal
    2  tablespoons minced fresh herbs
    2  teaspoons lemon juice

Sprinkle cod with lemon juice. Mix flour, cornmeal and herbs and dust the cod with the cornmeal-herb mixture. Bake in oven at 375 ºF for 10 minutes. Add salt and black pepper to taste.

<u>Serves 4</u>. One serving is about 230 Calories (for cod only).

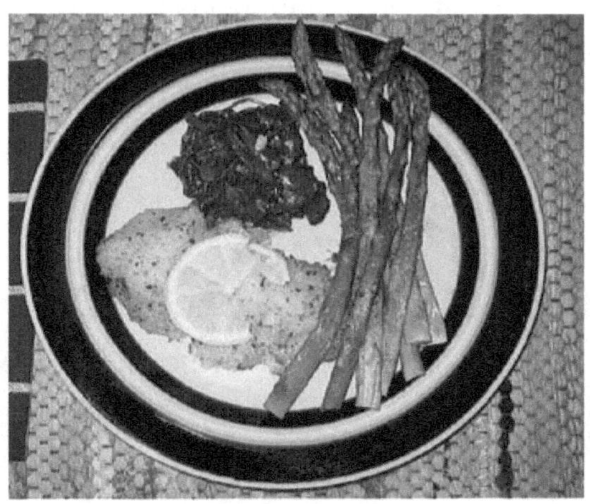

<u>Diet Tip of the Day:</u>. **A reducing diet is best supervised by a physician.** This is especially true when a great deal of weight needs to be lost, or if you have an ailment or a history of medical problems.

## Day 3 - French-Toast

   6 slices **GF bread***
   2 eggs
   ⅓ cup skim milk
   1 teaspoon vanilla
   A dash of cinnamon

In a medium bowl, beat together eggs and skim milk.  Add vanilla and cinnamon.  Saturate bread slices in egg mixture.  In a non-stick skillet coated with a **GF cooking oil spray** (page 123) cook bread slices until both sides are golden brown.  If desired, dust lightly with confectionary sugar.  Serve hot or keep in an oven or warmer at 200 °F until ready to plate.
**Serves 2**.  Three slices of French toast per serving.  Each serving is 310 Calories.

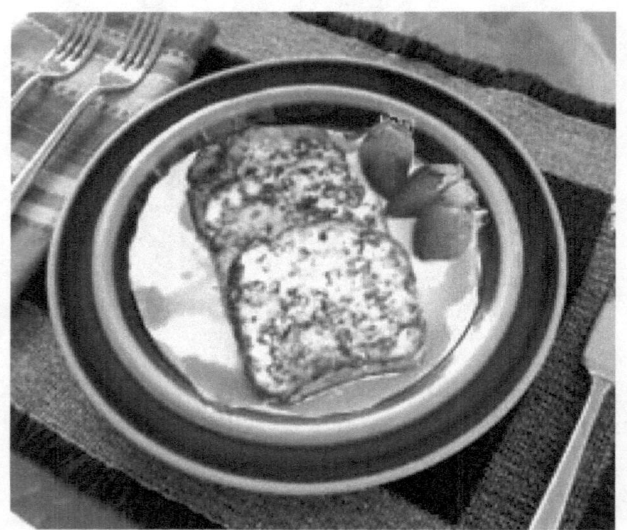

**Diet Tip of the Day:**  "Eat Slowly"  This is especially vital when you are trying to lose weight.  If you are someone who eats fast, who finishes before everyone else at the table, you are not giving yourself a chance to feel full.  While everyone else is still eating, you either sit there and pick, or you have seconds, taking in extra calories you could avoid if you would just slow down.

* We prepared this dish using Udi's gluten-free whole grain bread.  Delicious!

## <u>Day 4 - Carrie's Low-Cal Meat Loaf</u>

½ pound ground white meat turkey
½ pound ground beef (about 90% lean)
1 large egg
½ cup skim milk
¼ cup **GF bread crumbs** (page 117)
¼ cup ketchup
¼ cup chopped carrots
¼ cup chopped onion

In a medium bowl, combine all ingredients.  Add salt and pepper to taste.
Mix until blended and form into a loaf.  Place loaf into oven preheated to 350
°F.  Bake until an instant-read thermometer inserted in the center of the loaf
reads 160 °F.  This should take about one hour.

Shown below is meat loaf, acorn squash (baked with 1 teaspoon of pure
maple syrup).  Also shown is steamed spinach drizzled with extra-virgin
olive oil.

<u>Serves 5</u>.  About 290 Calories per serving (for meat loaf only).  Note: reserve
half a serving of the meat loaf which is to be eaten for lunch on Day 6.

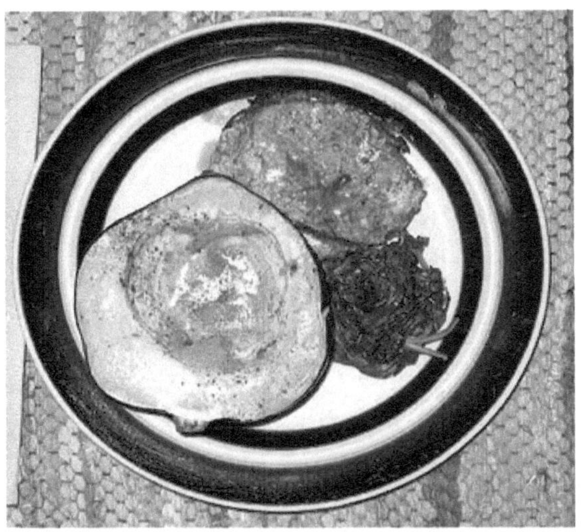

<u>Diet Tip of the Day:</u>  **Buy a pedometer** and start walking.  For the average
person 2,100 steps amounts to walking about one mile.  A Harvard study has
shown that 8,000 to 10,000 step per day promote weight loss.  And you're not
obliged to walk continuously until you accrue all 10,000 steps.  Rather, all
steps throughout the day to wherever and whenever count toward your daily
total steps

# Day 5 - Recipe

## Day 5 - Frozen Dinner

No recipe today.  No cooking today.  It's your day off!  At this writing, Amy's and Artisan Bistro offer quite a few gluten-free frozen entrees.  Smart Ones only makes two gluten-free entrees.  Glutino also makes two gluten-free frozen entrees, but both contain 400 Calories.

- Amy's Quinoa, Black Beans, Butternut Squash & Chard (**240 Cal**)
- Amy's Black Bean & Cheese Enchilada (**240 Cal**)
- Amy's Mushroom Risotto Bowl (**240 Cal**)
- Amy's Sweet & Sour Asian Noodle Bowl (**250 Cal**)
- Amy's Vegetable Parmesan Bowl (**260 Cal**)
- Amy's Brown Rice & Veggies Bowl – Light in Sodium (**260 Cal**)
- Amy's Brown Rice, Black-eyed Peas & Veggies Bowl (**290 Cal**)
- Amy's Teriyaki Bowl (**290 Cal**)
- Amy's Asian Noodle Stir Fry (**300 Cal**)
- Amy's Vegetable Lasagna (**300 Cal**)
- Amy's Thai Stir-Fry (**310 Cal**)
- Amy's Tofu Scramble (**320 Cal**)

- Artisan Bistro Wild Alaskan Salmon (**200 Cal**)
- Artisan Bistro Chicken Parmesan Bake (**200 Cal**)
- Artisan Bistro Turkey Cheddar Bake (**240 Cal**)
- Artisan Bistro Wild Alaskan Salmon Bake (**240 Cal**)
- Artisan Bistro Thai Style Yellow Curry with Chicken (**240 Cal**)
- Artisan Bistro Cheddar Beef Bake (**250 Cal**)
- Artisan Bistro Sesame Ginger with Salmon (**270 Cal**)
- Artisan Bistro Coconut Lemongrass with Chicken (**270 Cal**)
- Artisan Bistro Spiced Chicken Morocco (**270 Cal**)
- Artisan Bistro Albacore Tuna Bake (**280 Cal**)
- Artisan Bistro Thai Style Red Curry with Beef (**280 Cal**)
- Artisan Bistro Chicken Citron (**280 Cal**)
- Artisan Bistro Wild Alaskan Salmon with Pesto (**310 Cal**)
- Artisan Bistro Savory Turkey (**330 Cal**)
- Artisan Bistro Southwest Style Beef (**330 Cal**)
  - Artisan Bistro Ginger Chicken (**350 Cal**)
  - Artisan Bistro Beef with Mushroom Sauce (**350 Cal**)
  - Artisan Bistro Wild Alaskan Salmon Cake (**370 Cal**)

  - Smart Ones Lemon Herb Chicken Piccata (**250 Cal**)
  - Smart Ones Santa Fe Style Rice & Beans (**290 Cal**)

That's it.  There are just not many low-calorie frozen GF entrees currently in stores.  But  more food manufacturers are getting on the GF band wagon, so check your local supermarket for the latest gluten-free frozen entrees.  Also note that **340 Calories are allocated for this meal**.  But almost all of the above have less than 340 Calories.  Use the excess calories anyway you wish.  Splurge on extra dessert or save the calories for another day!

And please read the important **Frozen-Food Safety Warning** in **Appendix D** - page 226.

<u>**Diet Tip of the Day:**</u>   **Take a daily multi-vitamin/mineral supplement.**  This is important when you're on a reducing diet – as a kind of insurance policy.

## <u>Day 6 - Margherita Pizza</u>

In the original 30-Day Quick Diet we featured a pizza recipe used by Gail Johnson's Italian grandmother.  From feedback, our readers thought it was absolutely delicious - they loved it.  We tried hard to make the pizza gluten free but just couldn't get the same crust and taste.  After testing several commercially available brands of gluten-free pizza crust and finally settled on the following recipe (which makes two 9-inch pizzas):

    1   medium onion, minced & 1 clove of garlic, minced
    ¼   teaspoon dry oregano & ⅓.cup fresh basil leaves, torn
    3   oz part-skim mozzarella cheese, shredded
    2½ cups whole peeled canned tomatoes (page 118).
    1   tablespoon extra-virgin olive oil, divided
    2   9-inch diameter GF pizza crust*

<u>Tomato Sauce</u>: Over medium high heat, sauté minced onion in two teaspoons of olive oil.  Then stir in garlic, oregano, salt and pepper and ¼ teaspoon crushed red pepper (optional)..  Add tomatoes including most of the juice in the can, crushing them as you put them in pan.  Add ½ cup of water and simmer until sauce is reduced by one-half.

Brush one side of pizza crust with about a teaspoon of olive oil.  Spread tomato sauce over  crust and sprinkle shredded mozzarella cheese on top.  Place pizza on the lower rack of an oven preheated to 375°F.  Cook approximately 15 minutes or until cheese melts and bottom of pizza crust is brown.  Sprinkle with fresh basil leaves.  Cut and serve.

<u>Serves 4</u>.  230 Calories per serving.  One full pizza shown below but a serving is half of a pizza.

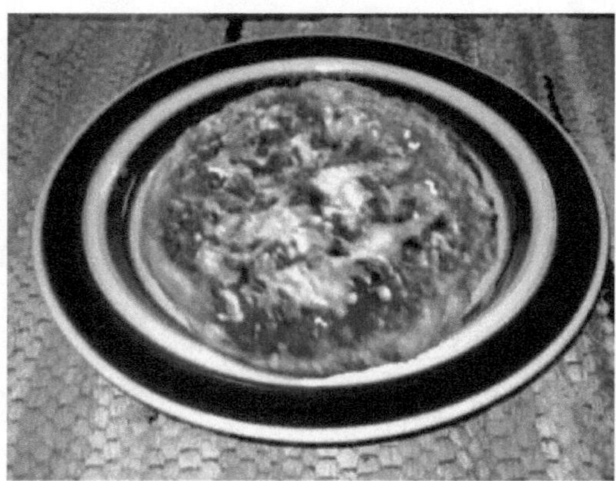

* We used Udi's GF Pizza Crust - 8 oz pkg which contains two 9-inch pizza crusts.

## <u>Day 7 - Chicken Dinner - Out</u>

No recipe today.  No cooking today.  Today you eat at a restaurant.  But when you are on a gluten-free reducing diet, eating in a restaurant can be a double challenge.  First, most restaurant portions are huge, easily totaling more than 1,000 Calories, and then many restaurants do not offer gluten-free menu selections.  On the *30-Day Gluten-Free Quick Diet*, a dinner type (i.e., fish, chicken, etc) and a calorie target are specified.  For example Day 7 of the 1,200 Calorie diet calls for a chicken dinner and allows you 530 Calories for appetizer, soup, main course and dessert.  Follow these tips to make sure your dinning experience is low calorie, gluten-free and pleasant.

Make sure you choose a restaurant where gluten-free food is available and where you have a fighting chance to achieve your calorie goal.  Before you out go read the menu online and reduce your food choices so you can have more focused questions for the staff.  You are more likely to get a safe meal if you call the restaurant before you go to let them know of your gluten-free needs.  And call during a slow time so you can have the host's complete attention.

In the restaurant, to ensure you are served a gluten-free meal, it is important to communicate your need to eat 100 percent gluten-free assertively but amiably. Try to speak directly to the chef or manager. Otherwise, ask your server what is in the food and how it is prepared. Menu descriptions do not always list every ingredient. Inquire how gluten-free grains such as rice and risottos are cooked. Sometimes they are cooked in broth which may contain gluten. Confirm that separate, clean utensils and equipment will be used to prepare your meal.

Order something simple, such as skinless white meat broiled chicken breast with steamed vegetables and brown rice.  Tell the waiter you want no sauce, no gravy, nothing added.  Then, knowing your calorie objective, and that most fish and chicken are about 50 Calories per ounce, most steamed vegetable servings average approximately 50 Calories per cup, and rice is about 100 Calories per ½ cup, decide how much to eat – and take the remainder home.  And consider bringing your own gluten-free salad dressing to the restaurant.  If fresh fruit is not an option, pass on dessert and have the evening snack specified in the *30-Day Gluten-Free Quick Diet* meal plan for that day.

In a restaurant, most nutritionists recommend you eat the low-calorie items on your plate first.  Start with the salad, soup and veggies.  By the time you get to the chicken and starches you will hopefully be full enough to be content with smaller portions of the higher-calorie choices.  (Incidentally, feel free to substitute skinless white meat turkey for chicken.)

We know that some dieticians advise their dieting clients not to eat out. They believe eating at home is safer.  But our thought is you have to eat out eventually so why not learn how while your resolve is high?

**Diet Tip of the Day:**  When you are on a diet and eating in a restaurant, a good rule of thumb is to **eat half of your entrée and bring the remainder home**.

## Day 8 - Baked Salmon with Salsa

This is a simple, straight-forward recipe.  The advantage of a simple recipe is there are no hidden calories.

    4   5 oz salmon fillets
    6   tablespoons bottled salsa*

Brown salmon fillets in non-stick pan and then place them in a baking dish. Cook fillets in an oven preheated to 350 ºF for about 10 minutes.  Plate the salmon.  Stir bottled tomato-pepper salsa and spoon it over the salmon. **Serves 4**.  One salmon fillet is about 215 Calories.

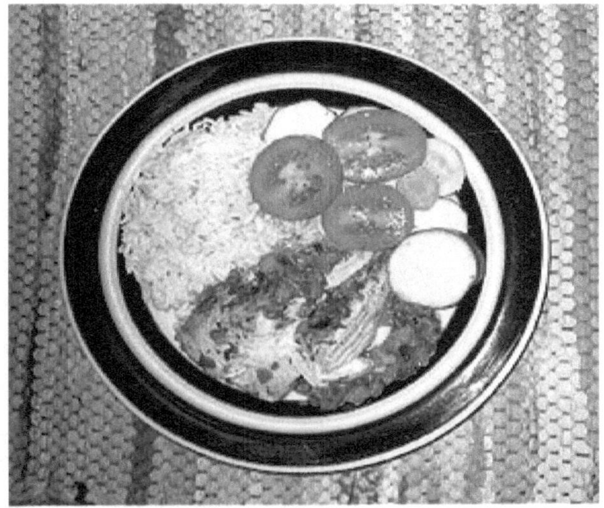

* We used Ortega's Garden Vegetable gluten-free salsa.  See page 119 for other gluten-free salsas.

**Diet Tip of the Day:** Hunger is your body's way of telling you that you need calories. But **when you're done eating, you should feel better – satisfied but not stuffed**.

## <u>Day 9 - Veggie Burger</u>

Vegetable-based burgers can be purchased at your local supermarket.  Patties of a veggie burger are made from either vegetables, soy, nuts, mushrooms, textured vegetable protein, dairy, or a combination of these foods.

Amy's makes two GF veggie burgers and Dr Paeger's makes one gluten free burger.  Amy's GF Bistro Veggie Burger is made with organic, brown rice, pinto beans, plenty of mushrooms and barbeque sauce (110 Calories per patty).  Amy's GF Sonoma Veggie Burger is made with organic vegetables, mushrooms and quinoa (140 Calories per patty).  Dr Praeger's GF California Veggie Burger is made with lots of organic vegetables (110 Calories per patty).

**Amy's Bistro Veggie Burger** patty shown below plus a slice of light GF cheese amounts to approximately 180 Calories.  The **GF bun** (see page 118) increases the total to 360 Calories.

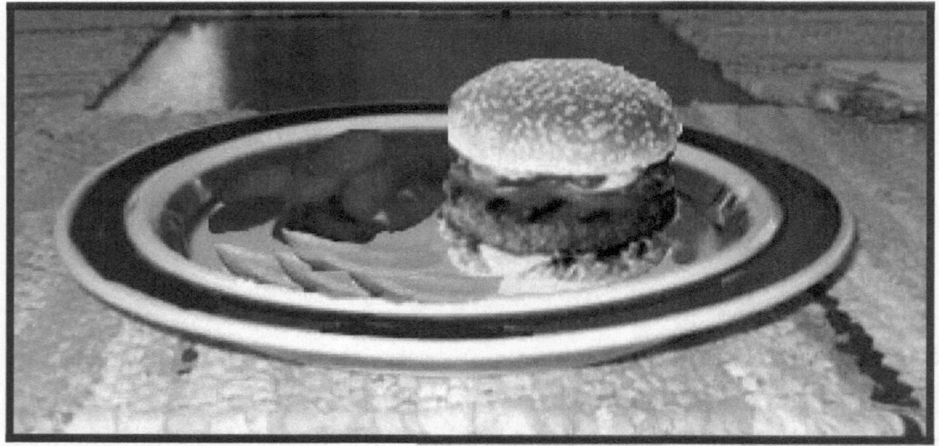

Photo shows seeded roll but most of the recommended GF burger rolls do not have seeds.

<u>Diet Tip of the Day:</u>  **Drink lots of water** – about 8 glasses per day when you're trying to lose weight.  Add a slice of lemon to make it more interesting.  Often, when you think you're hungry, you are just thirsty.  So, next time you crave a snack, drink some water first and see if that does it for you.

## <u>Day 6 - Wild Blueberry Pancakes</u>

This recipe makes a relatively low calorie, wholesome batch of delicious gluten-free wild blueberry buttermilk pancakes.

    1½ cups **gluten-free pancake mix** (page 117)
    1 cup buttermilk
    1 egg
    1 tablespoon vegetable oil

Stir ingredients until blended.  Add ¾ cup fresh of frozen blueberries and gently stir.  Let batter stand about 15 minutes for fluffier pancakes.

Using medium heat, preheat a non-stick skillet coated with cooking spray.  Pour slightly less than ¼ cup of batter onto skillet per pancake.  Cook slowly until bubbles break on surface of pancake.  Turn and cook until other side is golden brown.

Makes 8 pancakes about 4-inches in diameter.  Pictured below are two gluten-free blueberry pancakes with two slices of turkey bacon.

<u>Serves 4</u>.  Two pancakes per serving.  Each pancake is about 105 Calories

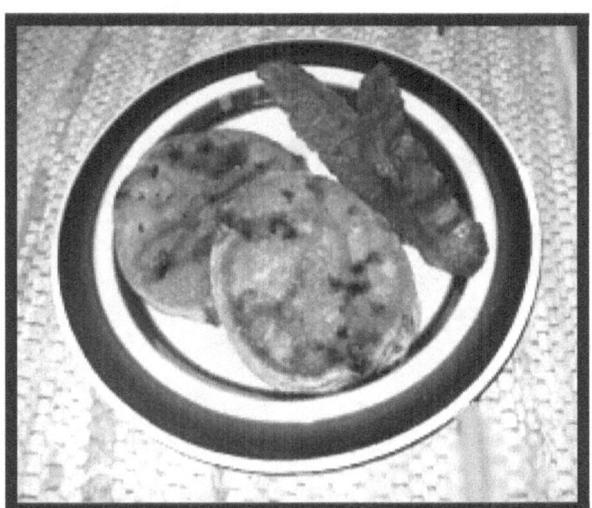

Bacon allowable only on 1,500 and 1,800 Calorie diets.

<u>**Diet Tip of the Day:**</u>  Most experts associate eating a substantial breakfast with successful weight loss.

## Day 11 - Artichoke-Bean Salad

    19-ounce can white kidney beans*
    10 artichoke hearts*, quartered
    ⅓ cup chopped oregano
    ⅓ cup chopped parsley
    3 cloves garlic, chopped
    1 lemon, juiced

Combine ingredients in medium-size bowl.  Stir in ¼ cup extra-virgin olive oil.  Salt and black pepper to taste.

**Serves 6**.  Approximately 190 Calories per serving.

Pictured on the plate below is the artichoke-bean salad as a side dish with two grilled chicken sausage links, tomato salsa and steamed green beans. Incidentally, this artichoke-bean combination over mixed salad greens served with a whole-grain bread makes a delicious, nutritious and reasonable low calorie main course.

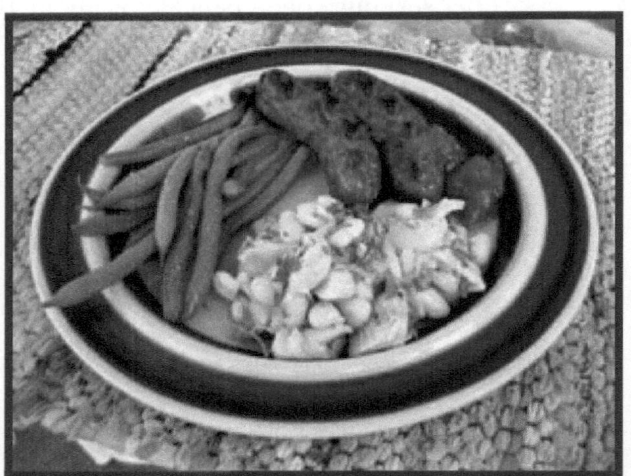

* Canned kidney beans and artichoke hearts should be gluten free but check the ingredients on the container to be sure.  Call the manufacturer and ask if the food product could contain trace gluten or could have been cross contaminated at their factory.  Do not eat a food if you are not sure it is gluten free.  Remember, if in doubt, go without.

**Diet Tip of the Day:**  Before you go to a **party**, have a small meal, such as a hardboiled egg, an apple, and a thirst quencher (like water, tea, seltzer, or diet soda).  This will take the edge off your appetite and make it easier to resist the high-calorie goodies.

# Day 12 - Recipe

## Day 12 - Fish Dinner - Out

No recipe today.  No cooking today.  Have a fish dinner at a restaurant, but make sure you choose a restaurant where you have a good chance to eat gluten free and achieve your calorie goal.  For today, your **goal for dinner is a maximum of 595 Calories**.  This includes appetizer, soup, main course and dessert.

**Tips for Eating Fish Out:**  The following is almost an exact repeat of the advice given eating out on previous days.  First make sure you choose a restaurant where gluten-free food is available and where you have a good chance to achieve your calorie goal.  Before you out go read the menu online and reduce your food choices so you can have more focused questions for the staff.  You are more likely to get a safe meal if you call the restaurant before you go to let them know of your gluten-free needs.  And call during a slow time so you can have the host's complete attention.

In the restaurant, to ensure you are served a gluten-free meal, it is important to communicate your need to eat 100 percent gluten-free assertively but pleasantly. Try to speak directly to the chef or manager. Otherwise, ask your server what is in the food and how it is prepared. Menu descriptions do not always list every ingredient. Inquire how gluten-free grains such as rice and risottos are cooked.  Sometimes they are cooked in broth which may contain gluten. Confirm that separate, clean utensils and equipment will be used to prepare your meal.

Order simple, such as broiled fish with steamed vegetables and brown rice.  Tell the waiter you want no sauce, no gravy, nothing added.  Then, knowing your calorie objective, and that fish is about 50 Calories per ounce, most steamed vegetable servings average approximately 50 Calories per cup, and rice is about 100 Calories per ½ cup, decide how much to eat – and take the remainder home.  And consider bringing your own gluten-free salad dressing to the restaurant.  If fresh fruit is not an option, pass on dessert and have the evening snack specified in the *30-Day Gluten-Free Quick Diet* meal plan for that day.

In a restaurant, most nutritionists recommend you eat the low-calorie items on your plate first.  Start with the salad, soup and veggies.  By the time you get to the chicken and starches you will hopefully be full enough to be content with smaller portions of the higher-calorie choices.

<u>**Diet Tip of the Day:**</u> Phytonutrients are found in plant foods such as fruits, vegetables, whole grains, dried beans, nuts and seeds.  Unlike protein, fat, vitamins and minerals, phytonutrients are not necessary for life, but evidence is growing that phytonutrients have many beneficial qualities.

91

## <u>Day 13 - Pasta with Marinara Sauce</u>

The spiral pasta profile shown below is called fusilli, a very popular pasta shape because all those ridges hold lots of tomato sauce.

  ½ small onion, finely chopped
  1 teaspoon olive oil
  2 garlic cloves, finely chopped
  1½ cups chopped plum tomatoes
  ½ teaspoon chopped fresh oregano
  ½ pound gluten-free fusilli pasta*
  ¼ teaspoon salt

**Homemade Tomato sauce:**  Sauté chopped onion in 1 teaspoon olive oil. Add two finely chopped garlic cloves, 1½ cups chopped plum tomatoes and ½ teaspoon chopped fresh oregano.  Stir and cook about 5 minutes on a low flame.

**Pasta**: Bring 2 quarts of lightly salted water to a boil.  Add GF pasta and stir occasionally (to keep pasta from sticking to the bottom of the pot).  Keep water boiling and cook until pasta are "al dente."  (Cooking time is about 9 minutes.)  Because the tomato sauce is a bit too thick, add ¼ cup of pasta liquid to the sauce to thin it.  Finally drain the pasta, add the marinara sauce and serve hot.

<u>Serves 4.</u>  One serving is about 250 Calories.

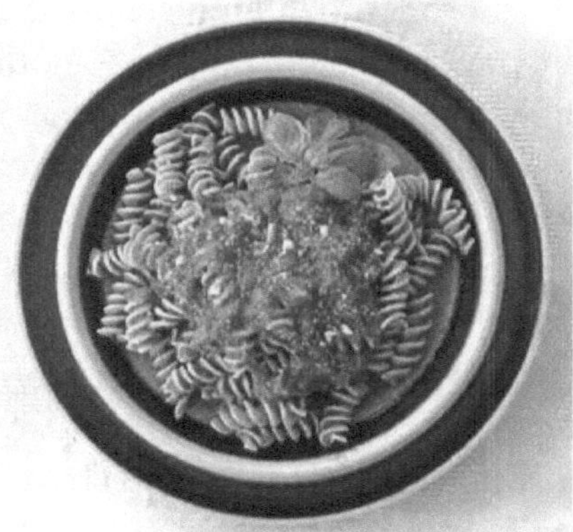

* We used Delallo Whole Grain Rice Fusilli.  Chef, Gail Johnson said, "DeLallo pasta is very good with a nice bite and an agreeable flavor."  See page 123 for additional gluten-free pasta choices.

<u>Diet Tip of the Day:</u>  **Beware of alcoholic beverages**.  Beer has about 13 Calories per ounce, wine 25 Calories per ounce and whiskey a whopping 71 Calories per ounce.

## Day 14 - Low-Cal Smoothie

Smoothies are delicious, nutritious and fun to drink!  They're great for a fast but nutritious breakfast, a light energy-boosting lunch, a healthy snack, a late afternoon pick me up, and a delicious dessert.  Making your own smoothie is a smart way to save money and get healthy at the same time!

    6 ounces GF plain non-fat **yogurt** (page 123)
    1 cup orange juice
    1 cup strawberries
    ¾ cup blueberries
    1 banana
    1 teaspoon sugar
    1 teaspoon vanilla extract

Place yogurt, strawberries, and blueberries in a blender.  Pour in orange juice. Add sugar and vanilla extract to mixture.  Blend all ingredients until thick and smooth.  Pour smoothie into a glass and enjoy.
**Serves 2**.  About 220 Calories per serving

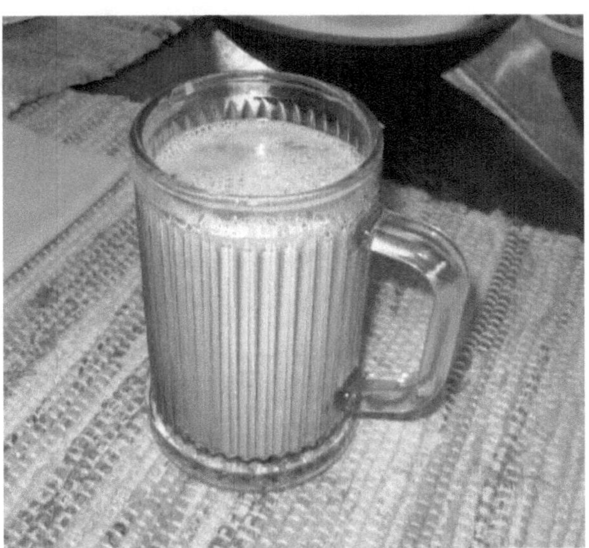

**Diet Tip of the Day:**  Two scientific journals indicate **dark chocolate** - not white chocolate or milk chocolate - is potent antioxidant and is good for you. But don't overdo it, because you have to offset the extra chocolate calories by eating less of other foods.

## <u>Day 15 - London Broil</u>

    1 lb boneless flank steak about ¾" thick, fat trimmed
    1 clove garlic
    1 teaspoon dry oregano (See **spices** page 119))

Rub each side of the flank steak with garlic.  Season with oregano, salt and pepper to taste.  Prepare a large non-stick skillet over high heat.  Steak should sizzle when placed on hot skillet.  Sear steak on one side for about 5 minutes; then turn and sear other side for about 4 minutes, or until done to preference.  Check the center by making small incision.  Carve into ¼-inch slices.
<u>Serves 4</u>.  About 320 Calories per serving (for meat only).

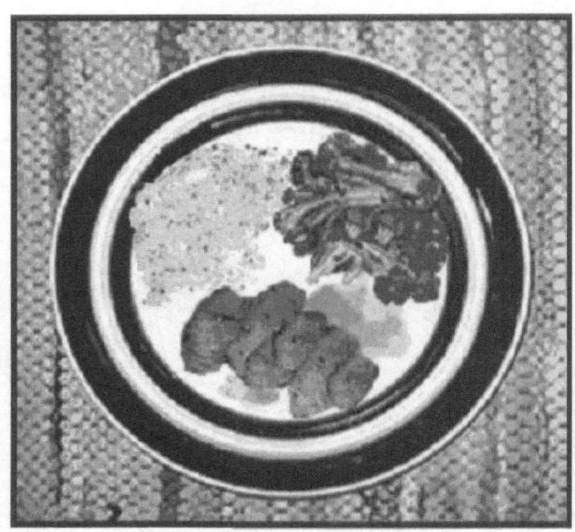

<u>**Diet Tip of the Day:**</u> **Stay Busy.**  Most people will do anything to avoid work, housework, yard work, exercise, etc.  But any kind of work burns a lot more calories than just sitting!  Whatever it is you are avoiding – just go do it!

## Day 16 - Recipe

## <u>Day 16 - Red Snapper with Special Sauce</u>

    4  4-ounce red snapper fillets (salmon fillets also okay)
    ½ cup white wine
    ½ cup plain GF plain non-fat **yogurt** mixed with ¼ cup mustard
    ½ pound green beans
    ¾ pint cherry tomatoes (about 20), halved
    4 teaspoons olive oil
    ¾ cup wild rice and brown rice mix.

Brown fillets in non-stick pan.  Place fillets skin side down in baking dish coated with non-stick spray.  Add white wine and cook in oven preheated to 350 ºF for about 15 minutes. Spoon pan juices over fillets.  Salt and pepper to taste.

Place green beans in skillet.  Add ¼-inch of water and cook over medium heat until water boils off.  Add cherry tomatoes and olive oil.  Stir well and sauté for a few minutes.  (If desired, season with fresh rosemary and oregano.)  Salt and pepper to taste.

Prepare rice mix per package directions.  Rice is naturally gluten free but check to make sure the rice mix you use is gluten-free.

Plate red snapper fillet and spoon over yogurt-mustard sauce.  Add green beans and tomato mix and the wild rice mix.  Serve hot.
**<u>Serves 4.</u>**  One plate consisting of one snapper fillet (215 Calories) with green beans and tomato mix (75 Calories) and wild rice (160 Calories) totals 450 Calories.

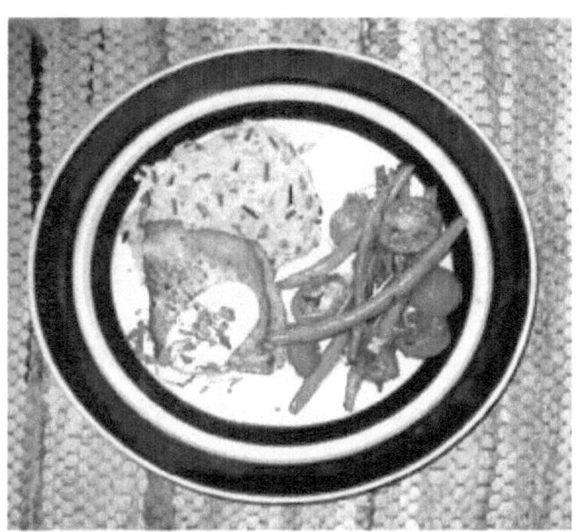

**<u>Diet Tip of the Day:</u>**  **Don't have sweets in your house**. This makes them easier to resist.  Out of sight, out of mind!

## Day 17 - Cajun Chicken Salad

This is a perfect after-work, quick, nutritious and delicious dinner.

    4 boneless and skinless chicken breasts - about 5 oz each

    4 teaspoons of bottled GF **Cajun herb-spice** mix (page 119)

    8 ounces mixed salad greens

    ¾ pint cherry tomatoes (about 20), halved

    12 pitted black olives

    2 tablespoons bottled light GF **salad dressing** (page 124)

Brush chicken breasts lightly with olive oil.  Roll breasts in Cajun herb-spice mix.

Brown breasts on non-stick oven-proof skillet.  After breasts are brown, put skillet in 350 ºF oven for approximately 15 minutes, or until done.  (When the breasts are done, the meat should be moist and white with no sign of pink.)  Cut breasts into ½-inch slices.

Serve hot or keep in an oven or warmer at 200 ºF until ready to plate.  Place chicken slices over a bed of mixed salad greens.  Add tomatoes, olives and two tablespoons of your favorite light GF salad dressing.

**Serves 4**.  330 Calories per serving

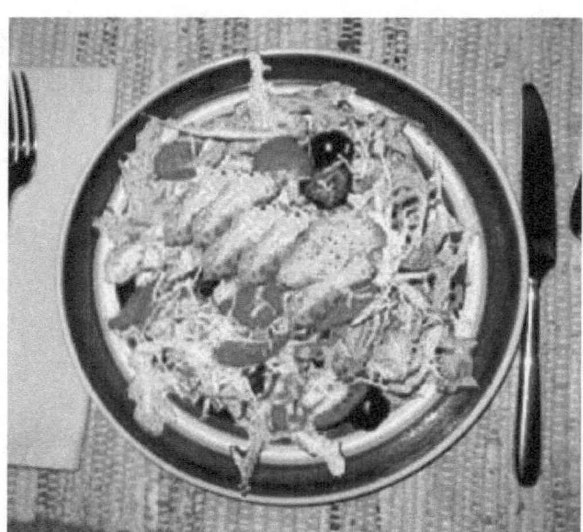

**Diet Tip of the Day:**  Hot or cold cereal topped with fruit, and fat-free milk makes a nutritious, relatively low-calorie meal anytime.

## <u>Day 18 - Grilled Swordfish</u>

  1¼ pounds swordfish
  ¾ pint cherry tomatoes (about 20), halved
  4 medium potatoes
  2 cups fresh spinach
  1 teaspoon rosemary & juice of ¼ lemon
  2 teaspoon extra-virgin olive oil, divided

Steam spinach with garlic and drizzle with about 1 teaspoon extra-virgin olive oil.

Cut potatoes in medium-size pieces and sprinkle with lemon juice, add rosemary, salt and black pepper. Place potatoes on grill for about 10 minutes, turning occasionally.

Toss cherry tomatoes in remaining extra-virgin olive oil. Add fresh oregano, salt and black pepper. Place on heavy-duty aluminum foil, seal and grill for about 3 minutes.

<u>GF Lemon-Herb Marinade</u>: 1 lemon - juiced, 1 Tbsp olive oil, 2 garlic cloves minced, 1 tsp fresh thyme chopped, 1 tsp fresh oregano chopped and 1 tsp minced green onion.

Immerse swordfish in GF marinade. Grill on hot fire for about 5 minutes on one side and 3 minutes on the other, or until done as desired.
**Serves 4**. One plate of grilled swordfish (250 Calories) with potatoes (100 Calories), cherry tomatoes (45 Calories) and steamed spinach (50 Calories) totals 445 Calories.

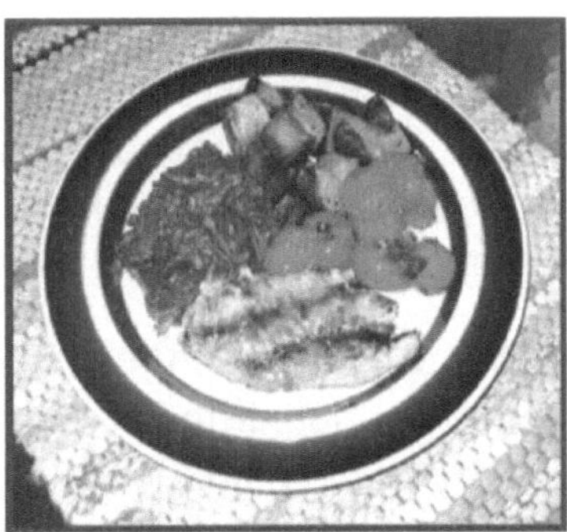

<u>**Diet Tip of the Day:**</u> **Slow weight loss is healthier**, is more likely to be permanent and is easier to sustain over the long haul. When it comes to weight loss, don't be in a hurry!

# Day 19 - Recipe

## Day 19 - Chinese Dinner - Out

No recipe today.  No cooking today.  Have a Chinese dinner at your favorite restaurant, but make sure you choose a restaurant where you can eat gluten free and have a reasonable chance to achieve your calorie goal.  For today, **your goal for dinner is a maximum of 640 Calories**.  This includes any appetizer, soup, main course and any dessert.

**Tips for Eating Chinese:**  Try bringing a restaurant card to the Chinese restaurant. The cards are available online and are designed to help explain a gluten-free diet to a waiter who might not speak English.

You can consume a lot of calories in a Chinese restaurant – if you order carelessly.  For example a typical portion of General Tso's chicken is loaded with about 1,000 Calories, then add another 200 Calories for a cup of rice.

First rule, order simple. Rice noodles prepared with vegetables or chicken are generally a safe choice. Avoid brown sauce which may have a soy sauce base. Instead, ask for the dish to be prepared with a white sauce using corn starch.  Then, knowing your 640 Calorie objective, and that chicken and fish are about 50 Calories per ounce, most steamed vegetable servings average approximately 50 Calories per cup, and rice is about 200 Calories per cup, decide how much of the meal you can eat – and take the remainder home.  (Note that you will be eating half a serving of left over Chinese food for lunch tomorrow.)  To stay within your maximum allowable calorie total, you should pass on dessert and have the evening snack (if any) specified for that day in the diet.

And although it is customary to share dishes at a Chinese restaurant, do not permit your dinner companions to contaminate your food. Make sure your friends do not use their gluten-contaminated spoons to serve food from your gluten-free dish.

Incidentally, although Chinese is specified, feel free to substitute Thai food, Vietnamese, Indian, Middle Eastern, or any other favorite ethnic food. Just make sure you can eat gluten free and do not exceed the maximum allowable 640 calories for this meal.

**Diet Tip of the Day:**  Another dilemma for dieters is **judging portion size**. It makes no sense to worry about whether to apportion 70 or 80 Calories per ounce for a cut of lean meat if you have no idea whether the portion you are planning to eat weighs four or ten ounces.  To be successful, you must learn to estimate portion sizes with reasonable accuracy.

## <u>Day 20 - Quick Pasta alla Puttanesca</u>

This famous pasta dish originated in Naples Italy. Puttanesca means "ladies of the night." Although the exact origin of the name is unclear, one thing is clear: It's delicious! Here is one of many recipe versions.

- ½ pound **GF spaghetti** (page 123)
- 20 black or green pitted olives
- 14.5-oz can diced tomatoes
- 4 oz GF **tomato sauce.** (page 119)
- 2 tablespoon extra-virgin olive oil
- 3 cloves of garlic, chopped
- 1 tablespoon dried minced onion
- ½ teaspoon crushed red pepper flakes
- 1 tablespoon capers drained and rinsed
- ¼ cup currants

Cook spaghetti according to package directions. Drain and return spaghetti to pot; add a teaspoon extra-virgin olive oil and toss to coat.

Heat remaining olive oil in large skillet over medium-high heat. Add red pepper flakes; cook and stir 1 to 2 minutes or until sizzling. Add onion and garlic; cook and stir 1 minute. Add canned tomatoes with juice, tomato sauce, olives, currants and capers. Cook over medium-high heat, stirring frequently, until sauce is heated through.

**<u>Serves 4</u>.** About 345 Calories per serving

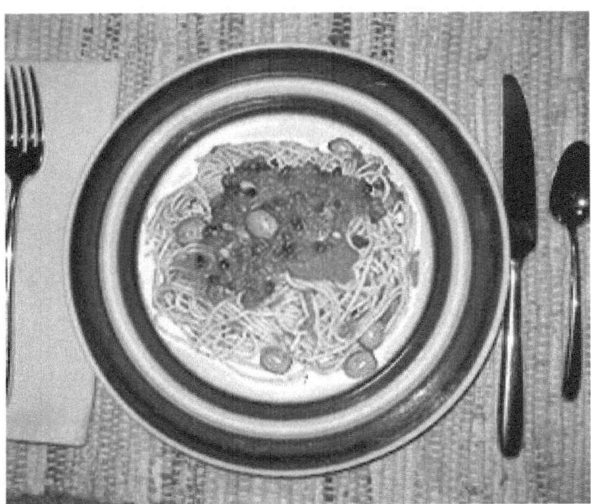

**<u>Diet Tip of the Day:</u>** Dilute fruit juices, such as apple juice, orange, etc. with water. This cuts the flavor slightly but really reduces calorie content.

# Day 21 - Recipe

## Day 21 - Frozen Dinner

No recipe today.  No cooking today.  It's your day off!  At this writing,
Amy's and Artisan Bistro offer quite a few gluten-free frozen entrees.
SmartOnes only makes two gluten-free entrees

- Amy's Quinoa, Black Beans, Butternut Squash & Chard (**240 Cal**)
- Amy's Black Bean & Cheese Enchilada (**240 Cal**)
- Amy's Mushroom Risotto Bowl (**240 Cal**)
- Amy's Sweet & Sour Asian Noodle Bowl (**250 Cal**)
- Amy's Vegetable Parmesan Bowl (**260 Cal**)
- Amy's Brown Rice & Veggies Bowl – Light in Sodium (**260 Cal**)
- Amy's Brown Rice, Black-eyed Peas & Veggies Bowl (**290 Cal**)
- Amy's Teriyaki Bowl (**290 Cal**)
- Amy's Asian Noodle Stir Fry (**300 Cal**)
- Amy's Vegetable Lasagna (**300 Cal**)
- Amy's Thai Stir-Fry (**310 Cal**)
- Amy's Tofu Scramble (**320 Cal**)

- Artisan Bistro Wild Alaskan Salmon (**200 Cal**)
- Artisan Bistro Chicken Parmesan Bake (**200 Cal**)
- Artisan Bistro Turkey Cheddar Bake (**240 Cal**)
- Artisan Bistro Wild Alaskan Salmon Bake (**240 Cal**)
- Artisan Bistro Thai Style Yellow Curry with Chicken (**240 Cal**)
- Artisan Bistro Cheddar Beef Bake (**250 Cal**)
- Artisan Bistro Sesame Ginger with Salmon (**270 Cal**)
- Artisan Bistro Coconut Lemongrass with Chicken (**270 Cal**)
- Artisan Bistro Spiced Chicken Morocco (**270 Cal**)
- Artisan Bistro Albacore Tuna Bake (**280 Cal**)
- Artisan Bistro Thai Style Red Curry with Beef (**280 Cal**)
- Artisan Bistro Chicken Citron (**280 Cal**)
- Artisan Bistro Wild Alaskan Salmon with Pesto (**310 Cal**)
- Artisan Bistro Savory Turkey (**330 Cal**)
- Artisan Bistro Southwest Style Beef (**330 Cal**)
  - Artisan Bistro Ginger Chicken (**350 Cal**)
  - Artisan Bistro Beef with Mushroom Sauce (**350 Cal**)
  - Artisan Bistro Wild Alaskan Salmon Cake (**370 Cal**)

  - Smart Ones Lemon Herb Chicken Piccata (**250 Cal**)
  - Smart Ones Santa Fe Style Rice & Beans (**290 Cal**)

That's it.  There are just not many low-calorie frozen GF entrees currently in stores.  But  more food manufacturers are getting on the GF band wagon, so check your local supermarket for the latest gluten-free frozen entrees.  Also note that **340 Calories are allocated for this meal**.  But almost all of the above have less than 340 Calories.  Use the excess calories anyway you wish.  Splurge on extra dessert or save the calories for another day!  And please read the important **Frozen-Food Safety Warning** in **Appendix D** - page 226.

**Diet Tip of the Day:**  **Understanding  nutrition**  is not only vital for good health but also will help you control your weight over the long term.  For example, did you know that foods that are labeled an "excellent source" of a particular nutrient provide 20% or more of the Recommended Daily Value.  Whereas, foods that are a "good source" of a nutrient provide between 10 and 20% of the Recommended Daily Value.

## Day 22 - Shrimp & Spinach Salad

   2 pounds shrimp in shell
   ½ pound small green beans, trimmed
   ½ pound baby spinach leaves
   2 tablespoon lemon juice
   ¼ cup extra-virgin olive oil
   2 teaspoon minced fresh dill
   1 tablespoon minced green onion

To make vinaigrette, combine lemon juice, olive oil, dill, salt and black pepper to taste and whisk until blended.  Stir in minced onion and set aside. Steam green beans and set aside.

Peel, de-vein and butterfly shrimp.  Place shrimp in a bowl and add water to cover.  Add 1 teaspoon of salt, and let stand for 10 minutes.  Drain, rinse, drain again, and dry.  Arrange shrimp in broiling pan without a rack.  Brush shrimp with a little of the vinaigrette and place under preheated broiler, about 3 inches from heat.  Broil about 3 to 4 minutes, turning shrimp once, or until both sides turn pink.

Remove shrimp from broiler and add remaining vinaigrette and green beans to the broiling pan.  Stir to coat shrimp and beans with vinaigrette. Pour warm vinaigrette over spinach and toss quickly.  Plate the spinach and arrange shrimp and green beans on top.
**Serves 4**.  310 Calories per serving.

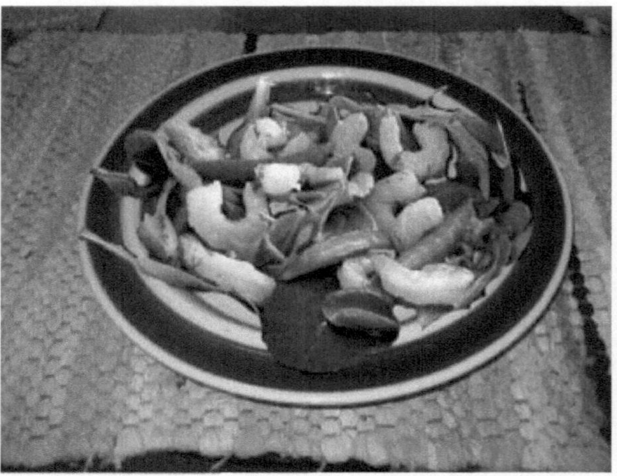

**Diet Tip of the Day:**  After company leaves, have them take some of the leftover food (particularly the dessert) with them – or take the leftovers to work the next day.

## <u>Day 23 - Beans & Greens Salad</u>

⅓ cup chopped oregano
⅓ cup chopped parsley
3 cloves garlic, chopped
1 lemon, juiced

Prepare dressing by combining above ingredients and stirring in ¼ cup extra-virgin olive oil.  Salt and black pepper to taste.

½ pound mesclun mix
¼ pound green beans
19-oz can garbanzo beans (chickpeas)*

Arrange mesclun mix, garbanzo beans and green beans on large platter.
Drizzle dressing over beans and greens.
<u>Serves 4</u>.  Approximately 260 Calories per serving.

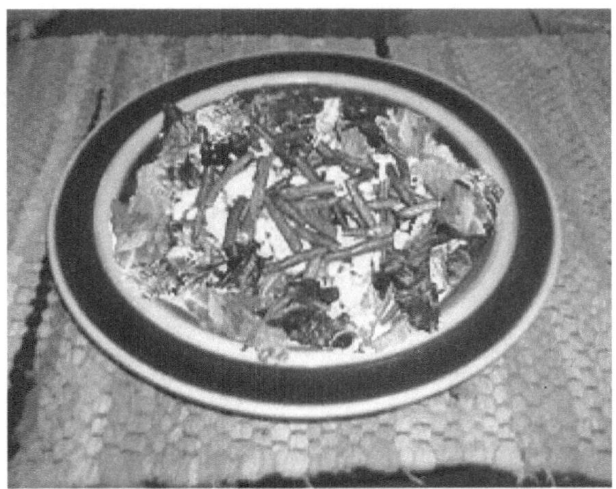

* Canned garbanzo beans should be gluten free but check the ingredients on the container to be sure.  Call the manufacturer and ask if the food product could contain trace gluten or could have been cross contaminated in their factory.  Do not eat a food if you are not sure it is gluten free.  Remember, if in doubt, go without.

<u>Diet Tip of the Day:</u>  Beans are a wonderful food but **beans are an incomplete protein**. If however beans are eaten with a whole-grain bread, the combination forms a complete protein – just as complete and nutritious as meat, poultry, or fish.

<h1 align="center">Day 24- Recipe</h1>

**<u>Day 24 - Four-Bean Plus Salad</u>**  (This is a side dish)

Note that the total caloric value of the salad will change very little, if the proportions of the bean varieties and corn are varied – according to taste. Make sure the canned foods are gluten free.

- ½ cup canned red kidney beans*, drained and rinsed
- ½ cup canned black beans*, drained and rinsed
- ½ cup canned chick peas*, drained and rinsed
- ½ cup canned cannelloni beans*, drained and rinsed
- ½ cup canned corn, drained
- 1 small red pepper, chopped
- 1 small green pepper, chopped
- 2 tablespoons extra-virgin olive oil
- 2 tablespoons lemon juice

In a large bowl mix red kidney beans, black beans, chick peas, cannelloni beans, corn and chopped red and green peppers.  Stir in olive oil and lemon juice and plate.

**<u>Serves about 6</u>**.  One serving is ½ cup – with about 135 Calories per serving

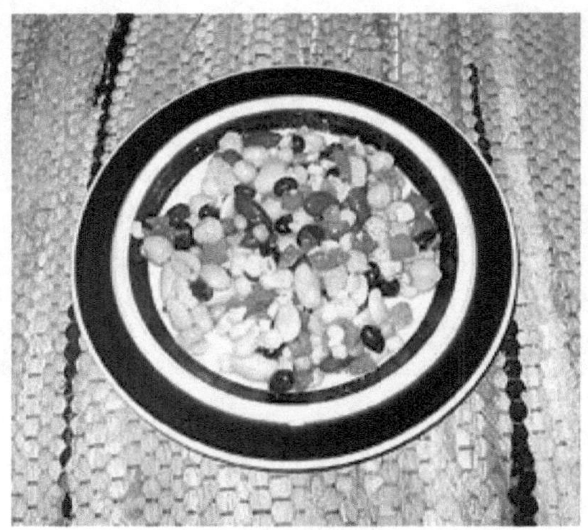

* Canned red kidney beans, black beans, chick peas and cannelloni beans should be gluten free but check the ingredients on the container to be sure.  Call the manufacturer and ask if the food product could contain trace gluten or could have been cross contaminated in their factory.  Do not eat a food if you are not sure it is gluten free.  Remember, if in doubt, go without.

**<u>Diet Tip of the Day:</u>** Vigorous exercise doesn't necessarily stimulate you to overeat. Just the opposite.  In many cases, exercise actually helps curb your appetite – immediately following a workout.

## <u>Day 25 - Pan-Broiled Hanger Steak</u>

   1¼ pounds hanger steak, well trimmed of fat
   ¼ cup lime juice
   8 small new potatoes, peeled and halved
   ½ pint cherry tomatoes (about 15), halved

Season both sides of steak with salt and pepper and place in sealable plastic bag with lime juice.  Refrigerate for about one hour.

Boil potatoes about 10 minutes.  Rinse in cold water.  Sauté potatoes in small amount of vegetable oil over medium-high heat until brown.

Sauté cherry tomatoes in small amount of olive oil over medium-high heat until skin begins to crack.  Season with chopped fresh basil.

Heat a skillet over medium-high heat.  Sear hanger steak on one side for about 5 minutes. Turn over and sear other side approximately 5 minutes (for medium done).  Pour off any fat that may have accumulated.  Cut into ½-inch slices.

<u>Serves 4.</u>  About 320 Calories per serving (for the hanger steak only)

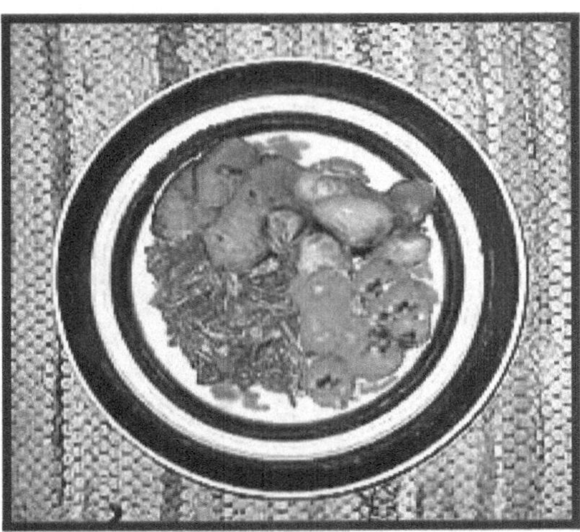

<u>Diet Tip of the Day:</u> If you go to a **party**, don't stand near the food!  Be aware of the temptation.  Make the effort, and you'll find you eat less.

## <u>Day 26 - Tina's Grilled Scallops &Polenta</u>

1 pound sea scallops
¾ cup GF **polenta** (page 117)
¾ cup skim milk
1 medium portobello mushroom
½ pound green beans
¼ cup chopped red onion
16 asparagus spears
1 teaspoon extra-virgin olive oil

Bring 1½ cups of water and skim milk to rapid boil.  Add salt to taste and slowly add GF polenta while stirring.  Reduce heat.  Continue stirring until desired consistency is reached.  Pour polenta into lightly greased pan.  After polenta has cooled cover and refrigerate.  Cut chilled polenta into 4 pieces.  Grill on medium-hot fire – about two minutes on each side.

Brush portobello mushroom and asparagus spears with olive oil and place on grill for about 3 minutes on each side.

Grill scallops on medium-hot fire.  Turn after two minutes or when first side turns opaque.  Grill until second side turns opaque – about another 2 minutes.  Don't overcook but test  a scallop by cutting to make sure it's cooked through.  Salt and pepper to taste.
<u>Serves 4.</u>  The food on the plate pictured below totals about 380 Calories.

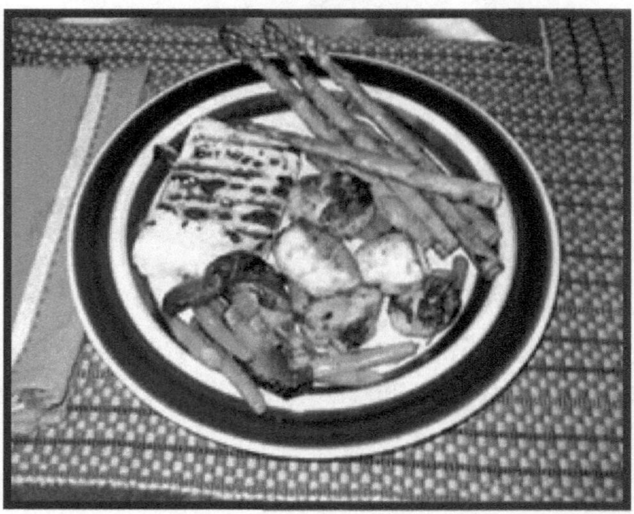

<u>Diet Tip of the Day:</u>  To have better control of what you eat **bring your lunch to work**.

## <u>Day 27 - Fettuccine in Summer Sauce</u>

This sauce is often served in the summer because it's lighter than what is usually dished up with pasta.  But despite its name the sauce is wonderful year round.

½ lb GF fettuccine pasta*

8 oz fresh asparagus, trimmed & cut in 2-inch pieces

¾ pint cherry tomatoes (about 20), halved

2 Tbsp plus 1 tsp extra-virgin olive oil, divided

2 cloves of garlic, chopped

½ small onion, diced

Cook GF fettuccine according to package directions.  Drain and return pasta to pot; add a teaspoon of the olive oil and toss to coat.  Meanwhile steam asparagus and drain.

In large skillet over medium-high heat, sauté cherry tomatoes in remaining 2 tablespoons of olive oil until skin begins to crack.  Add onion and cook until translucent.  Stir in garlic.  Thin sauce with pasta liquid to desired consistency.  Toss cooked pasta and asparagus into sauce and serve immediately.

<u>Serves 4</u>.  About 290 Calories per serving

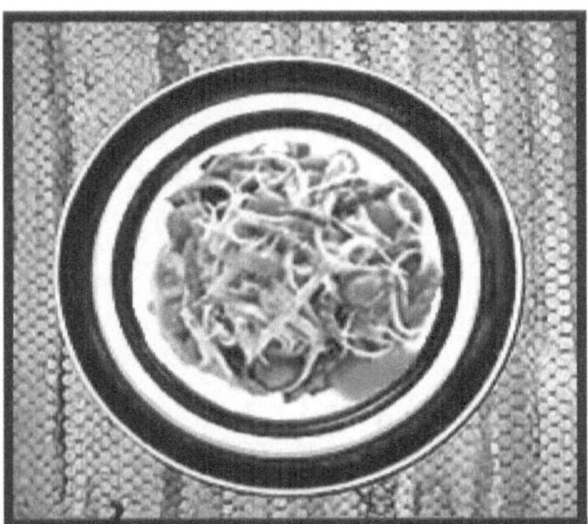

* If you cannot find gluten-free fettuccine, feel free to substitute any other shape of GF pasta.

<u>**Diet Tip of the Day:**</u>  A major weight-loss fallacy is that you can **get rid of abdominal fat** by working your abdominal muscles.  This is based on the incorrect belief that fat is eliminated from a particular part of your body if you engage the muscles underneath that layer of fat.  No such luck.

# Day 28 - Recipe

## Day 28 - Frozen Dinner

No recipe today.  No cooking today.  It's your day off!

- Amy's Quinoa, Black Beans, Butternut Squash & Chard (**240 Cal**)
- Amy's Black Bean & Cheese Enchilada (**240 Cal**)
- Amy's Mushroom Risotto Bowl (**240 Cal**)
- Amy's Sweet & Sour Asian Noodle Bowl (**250 Cal**)
- Amy's Vegetable Parmesan Bowl (**260 Cal**)
- Amy's Brown Rice & Veggies Bowl – Light in Sodium (**260 Cal**)
- Amy's Brown Rice, Black-eyed Peas & Veggies Bowl (**290 Cal**)
- Amy's Teriyaki Bowl (**290 Cal**)
- Amy's Asian Noodle Stir Fry (**300 Cal**)
- Amy's Vegetable Lasagna (**300 Cal**)
- Amy's Thai Stir-Fry (**310 Cal**)
- Amy's Tofu Scramble (**320 Cal**)

- Artisan Bistro Wild Alaskan Salmon (**200 Cal**)
- Artisan Bistro Chicken Parmesan Bake (**200 Cal**)
- Artisan Bistro Turkey Cheddar Bake (**240 Cal**)
- Artisan Bistro Wild Alaskan Salmon Bake (**240 Cal**)
- Artisan Bistro Thai Style Yellow Curry with Chicken (**240 Cal**)
- Artisan Bistro Cheddar Beef Bake (**250 Cal**)
- Artisan Bistro Sesame Ginger with Salmon (**270 Cal**)
- Artisan Bistro Coconut Lemongrass with Chicken (**270 Cal**)
- Artisan Bistro Spiced Chicken Morocco (**270 Cal**)
- Artisan Bistro Albacore Tuna Bake (**280 Cal**)
- Artisan Bistro Thai Style Red Curry with Beef (**280 Cal**)
- Artisan Bistro Chicken Citron (**280 Cal**)
- Artisan Bistro Wild Alaskan Salmon with Pesto (**310 Cal**)
- Artisan Bistro Savory Turkey (**330 Cal**)
- Artisan Bistro Southwest Style Beef (**330 Cal**)
  - Artisan Bistro Ginger Chicken (**350 Cal**)
  - Artisan Bistro Beef with Mushroom Sauce (**350 Cal**)
  - Artisan Bistro Wild Alaskan Salmon Cake (**370 Cal**)

- Smart Ones Lemon Herb Chicken Piccata (**250 Cal**)
- Smart Ones Santa Fe Style Rice & Beans (**290 Cal**)

**Diet Tip of the Day:**   **Take a daily multi-vitamin/mineral supplement.**  This is important when you're on a reducing diet – as a kind of insurance policy.

## <u>Day 29 - Barbequed Shrimp & Corn</u>

    1½ pounds large shrimp, peeled and de-veined
    3 Tbsp of bottled **GF barbeque sauce** (page 118)
    4 medium ears of corn

Pour barbeque sauce into shallow bowl. Toss shrimp in barbeque sauce to coat. Place shrimp on medium-hot grill. Turn shrimp after about two minutes or when shrimp turn pink. Grill until second side turns pink – approximately another 2 minutes. Don't overcook but test a shrimp by cutting to make sure it is cooked through. Salt and pepper to taste. Serve hot or at room temperature.

<u>Serves 4</u>. About 160 Calories per serving (shrimp only).

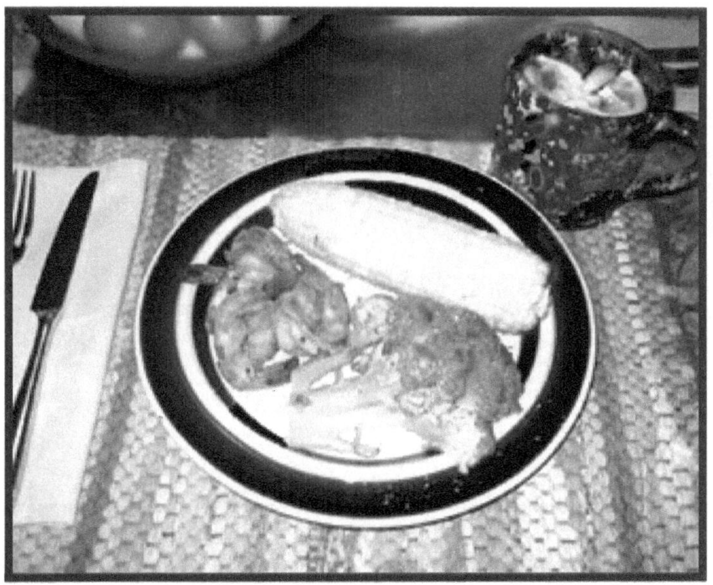

<u>**Diet Tip of the Day:**</u> A very **important weight-profile parameter** is your waist-to-hip ratio. Health risks for heart attack and stroke increase considerably for men with a ratio above 1.0 and for women with a ratio above 0.8. To calculate your ratio, measure your waist size (at its narrowest circumference) and divide it by your hip size (at the widest section).

## Day 30 - Cheeseburger Heaven

There's really not much to grilling hamburgers.  The ideal meat for a juicy burger is ground chuck with about 20% fat, but we are talking diet here.  So we opt for leaner, much leaner meat.

    1¼ pounds ground sirloin (95% lean)

    4 thin slices **light GF cheese** (page 123)

Mix ground beef in large bowl.  Salt and pepper to taste.  Divide into 4 equal portions and form burgers about 1-inch thick.

Cook burgers over a hot fire on charcoal or gas-fired grill.  For medium, cook about 4 minutes on each side.  Top with slice of light GF cheese.  Add lettuce and tomato.  Season to taste.

**Serves 4**.  About 320 Calories per serving (cheeseburger only).

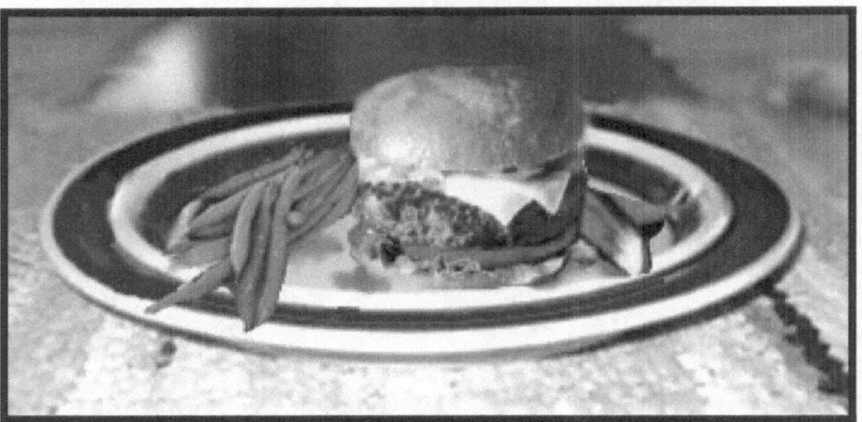

**Diet Tip of the Day:  Plan to be on a diet the rest of your life**.  Not necessarily a weight reducing diet.  At some point you'll want to just maintain your weight.  But you will still need to continue to make good healthy food choices – and not slip back to your old eating habits.

# Appendix A
# Gluten Notes

**Celiac Disease**:  The primary reason for a gluten-free diet is to combat celiac disease which is a chronic, systemic, autoimmune disorder that causes intestinal damage.  Common celiac symptoms include diarrhea, abdominal pain, weight loss and fatigue.  On the other hand, some celiac suffers experience constipation instead of diarrhea, weight gain instead of weight loss and heartburn instead of stomach pain.  And a few people diagnosed with celiac disease have almost no symptoms.  In net, celiac affects many body systems in different ways and because every person displays celiac disease differently, it is a difficult condition to diagnose.  A strict gluten-free diet most often alleviates celiac-related symptoms.  Keep in mind that all of these possible celiac disease symptoms can be caused by other medical problems.  If you suspect you have celiac disease, make sure to see a physician.

**Non Celiac Gluten Sensitivity**:  Another reason to go gluten free is to combat a condition called non-celiac gluten sensitivity that can also affect nearly every system in the body with symptoms that include digestive complaints, skin problems, brain fog, joint pain and numbness in extremities.  Because research into this condition is in its early stages, not all physicians have accepted it as an illness and as a result not all physicians provide patients with a diagnosis of gluten sensitivity.  Nevertheless, if you believe you suffer from gluten sensitivity, see a physician.  To make matters even more confusing, some people are allergic to wheat.  These people experience typical allergy symptoms (nasal congestion, etc) and sometimes they also have gastrointestinal symptoms.

**Healthier Way to Lose Weight**:  A new reason to go gluten free is that some medical practitioners believe it is a healthier way to lose weight.  But gluten-free weight loss is a recent concept and to date there has not been any research that confirms going gluten free promotes weight loss.  Many physicians, however, report a considerable number of their patients claim that when they went gluten free they lost weight and felt a lot better.

**Gluten Restriction Levels**:  Because people with celiac disease and gluten sensitivity have remarkably varying degrees of reaction to trace levels of gluten, it is useful to think in terms of three levels of gluten restriction:

The <u>first level</u> consists of adults with celiac disease.  These individuals have a medical reason for being on a gluten-free diet and have serious reactions to gluten.  They should avoid not only obvious gluten-laden foods, but also should avoid processed foods that have trace amounts of gluten as well as gluten-free foods that have been cross-contaminated by gluten foods or by trace gluten.  (The obvious gluten-laden foods include bread, cereals, and all products with wheat, barley or rye as an ingredient.)

The <u>second level</u> of gluten restriction consists of individuals with non-celiac gluten sensitivity or a wheat allergy who may or may not have a reaction to trace gluten in their food.  These people should avoid the obvious gluten containing foods and by trial and error learn what supposedly gluten-free foods (that nevertheless might contain trace gluten) they should also avoid.

In the <u>third level</u> are those who only want to lose weight and feel better on a gluten free diet.  These people have only to avoid obvious gluten-containing foods.

**Eating Gluten Free in Brief**:  First, you should be aware of food label ingredients that mean that gluten grains are present:  these are triticum vulgare (wheat), triticum spelta (a form of wheat), triticale (cross between wheat and rye), hordeum vulgare (barley) and secale cereale (rye).

Any of the following ingredients on a label indicate that the food definitely contains gluten: wheat protein, hydrolyzed wheat protein, wheat starch, hydrolyzed wheat starch, wheat flour, bread flour, bleached flour, bulgur (a form of wheat), malt (made from barley), couscous (made from wheat), farina (made from wheat), pasta (made from wheat unless otherwise indicated), seitan (made from wheat gluten and commonly found in vegetarian meals) and wheat germ oil or extract (likely cross contaminated).

Any of the following on a label indicate that the food might contain gluten: vegetable protein, hydrolyzed vegetable protein (could be from wheat, corn or soy), modified starch, modified food starch (can come from several sources, including wheat), natural flavor (can be made from barley), artificial flavor (can come from barley), modified food starch, hydrolyzed plant protein (HPP), hydrolyzed vegetable protein (HVP), seasonings, flavorings, vegetable starch, dextrin (sometimes made from wheat) and maltodextrin (sometimes made from wheat).

If a product contains wheat, the FDA requires that it be stated on the food's label. But other gluten-containing grains (barley or rye) do not have to be declared although they might have been added to a food's ingredients. If in doubt, check with the food manufacturer to determine if a food is truly gluten free. (Incidentally, when you call a manufacturer, it is not unusual for them to offer discount coupons for their products!)

**Gluten Cross Contamination**:  Of course, a food that has no gluten-containing ingredients could be cross contaminated with gluten.  For example, soybeans and oats do not naturally contain gluten.  But soybeans and oats are frequently grown in rotation with wheat crops. That means farmers often use the same fields to grow soy, oats  and wheat, they use the same combines to harvest the crops, the same storage facilities and the same trucks to transport the crops to market.  As a result, soy and oats are often gluten cross-contaminated.

So if you react to a food that is not supposed to have any gluten ingredients, it is probably because the food contains trace gluten due to cross contamination. The food might have just enough trace gluten to give you problems, despite having an apparently safe list of ingredients.

Appreciate that reactions to gluten vary from person to person. And a gluten reaction is influenced not only by how much gluten is in a food, but also by how much of that food you eat.

**Gluten-Free Labeling Standards**: The quantity of gluten in a particular product is expressed as parts of gluten contained in a million parts of the product, stated as parts per million, or ppm of gluten.  In 2013, the U.S. Food and Drug Administration allowed food manufacturers to label products "gluten-free" that contain less than 20 ppm of gluten (GF 20). Canada the UK and most European Union countries also consider 20 ppm to be gluten free. (20 ppm means a product contains 0.002% gluten).  Some people, however, still react to products labeled "gluten-free" that contain less than 20 ppm of gluten.  Because of this, several food manufacturers maintain more rigorous standards, typically lowering the amount of gluten in a product to less than 5 or 10 ppm.

# Appendix B
# Gluten-Free Foods

Because food ingredients and formulations can change at any time, the following lists and recommendations should only be used as a guide. Read the food label and ingredient statement on the food package carefully at the time of purchase to ensure it is gluten free.  Moreover, recall that only people with celiac disease and those with extreme gluten sensitivity usually need to be concerned with trace gluten.

And keep in mind our gluten-free guideline: "If in doubt, go without." Do not eat a supposedly gluten-free food if there is no ingredient list or if you are not sure whether the ingredients are gluten-free. If you are unsure of the ingredients, call the food manufacturer for more information.

Finally, although the following list is reasonably comprehensive, it does not contain all the gluten-free foods being sold.  And more gluten-free products are continually being developed and found on store shelves.

**Baking Mixes, etc**: Any baking mix you buy should be labeled "gluten-free." Most baking supplies, such as baking soda, sugar and cocoa, are considered gluten-free, but check ingredients to make certain. Davis, Rumford, Bob's Red Mill and Clabber Girl's baking powder are gluten free.
**All Purpose Flour**: Bob's Red Mill, King Arthur and other mills make gluten-free all-purpose flour.
**Corn Meal**:  Corn meal should be safe but check the label carefully.  Bob's Red Mill makes corn meal in gluten-free factory.
**Pancake Mix**: Bob's Red Mill, King Arthur, Bisquick and others make gluten free pancake mix.
**Pizza Dough**: Bob's Red Mill and King Arthur also make gluten free pizza dough.

**Bread Products**: The gluten in wheat, barley and rye consists of two proteins that combine during the baking process to form a substance that provides bread and other baked goods with elasticity and structure. Gluten also helps bread dough rise into a light, airy loaf.  Other grains do not have these characteristics, which is why it is difficult to find passable gluten-free bread. These days many supermarkets stock gluten-free bread, but you often can find a better selection online.
**Bread**: Udi's Whole Grain Bread (65 Calories per slice), Udi's White Sandwich Bread (70 Calories per slice) and Udi's Cinnamon Raisin Bread (70 Calories per slice), as well as many others are gluten free.
**Bread Crumbs**: Kinnikinnick Panko-Style Bread Crumbs are gluten free.

**Chow Mein Noodles**:  Goldberg's makes GF chow mein noodles.  They are sold in Walmart and many supermarkets.

**Hamburger Buns**: Kinnikinnick's Hamburger Buns (150 Calories), Rudi's Multi-Grain Hamburger Buns (190 Calories) and Udi's Classic and Whole-Grain Hamburger Buns (190 and 180 Calories per bun) are all gluten free.

**Hot Dog Buns**: Kinnikinnick's Hot Dog Buns (150 Calories), Rudi's Multi-Grain Hot Dog Buns (140 Calories) and Udi's Classic and Whole-Grain Hot Dog Buns (190 Calories) are all gluten free.

**Pita Bread**: Toufayan (110 Calories) sells gluten-free wraps.

**Polenta**: Bob's Red Mill Gluten Free Corn Grits/Polenta is gluten free.

<u>Cereals</u>: Some major brands now make several gluten-free cereals:
- General Mills Rice Chex (100 Calories per cup)
- General Mills Corn Chex (120 Calories per cup)
- General Mills Vanilla Chex (120 Calories per ¾ cup)
- General Mills Cinnamon Chex (120 Calories per ¾ cup)
- General Mills Chocolate Chex (130 Calories per ¾ cup)
- General Mills Apple Cinnamon Chex (130 Calories per ¾ cup)
- General Mills Honey Nut Chex (120 Calories per ¾ cup)
- Glutino Honey Nut (120 Calories per ¾ cup)
- Glutino Apple Cinnamon (120 Calories per ¾ cup).
- Kellogg's Rice Krispies - gluten-free (110 Calories per cup)
- Cream of Rice (150 Calories per packet)
- Bob's Red Mill Oat Meal
- GF Harvest Oat Meal (150 Calories per ½ cup)

- Waffles: Van's makes six varieties of gluten free waffles.

<u>**Coffee, Tea, Soda, Fruit Drinks and Alcohol**</u>: Unflavored coffee and black or green tea should be gluten-free, but flavored varieties may not be.  Most popular sodas in the United States are gluten-free.  Juice that is 100 percent fruit should be gluten-free, but fruit drinks made from fruit plus other ingredients may not be.  Conventional beer contains gluten; whereas, wine is gluten-free.

<u>**Condiments, Spices & Sauces**</u>: In most cases, you will need to check ingredients or call the manufacturer to determine whether their product is gluten free.

**BBQ sauces:** Sweet Baby Ray's BBQ Sauce (35 Calories per tablespoon any variety), and KC Masterpiece BBQ Sauce (30 Calories per tablespoon any variety) are gluten free.

**Cajun Herb-Spice Mix**: Cajun's Choice Blackened and Creole Seasoning, Cajun Quick Shake Seasonings and McCormick's Cajun Seasoning are gluten free.

**Herb's & Spices**: . Regular salt and pepper should be gluten-free. Fresh herbs and spices in a store's produce section are safe. McCormick's single ingredient spices are gluten-free to 20 parts per million and their spice blends like Italian Seasoning and Salad Supreme Seasoning are gluten free. Check other spice manufacturers for possible gluten cross-contamination.

**Marinades**: Bone Suckin' Original (also Poultry, Seafood & Steak) Seasoning & Rub and Kikkoman Gluten-Free Teriyaki Marinade & Sauce.

**Mustard & Ketchup**: French's yellow mustard and Heinz ketchup are gluten-free.

**Salsas:** The following salsas are gluten free to 20 ppm. All varieties have 5 to 8 Calories per tablespoon.
- Amy's Salsa (mild & medium)
- Amy's Black Bean & Corn
- Farmer's Garden Salsa (medium & hot)
- Farmer's Peach
- Farmer's Pineapple
- Farmer's Roasted Garlic
- Newman's Own Black Bean & Corn
- Ortega Black Bean & Corn
- Ortega Garden Vegetable
- Ortega Original
- Ortega Thick & Chunky
- Ortega Salsa Verde

**Soy Sauce**: San-J and Kikkoman make gluten-free soy sauce.

**Tomato Sauce**: The following tomato sauces are both gluten free and low calorie:
- Classico Tomato & Basil Sauce (90 Calories per cup)
- Prego Light Smart Italian Sauce (90 Calories per cup)
- Hunt's Tomato Sauces (80 Calories per cup).

**Tomato Paste**: Hunt's is gluten free.

**Canned Tomatoes**: Most canned tomatoes are safe including (but not limited to) Hunt's, Del Monte and Contadina.

**Vinegar:** Distilled vinegar is derived from gluten grains but usually tests below the 20 ppm gluten threshold and is generally considered safe. Quite a few people with celiac and gluten sensitivity, however, report that they react to both distilled vinegar and distilled alcohol. To be safe, look for cider or balsamic vinegar rather than distilled vinegar.

**Worcestershire Sauce**: Lea & Perrins and French's Worcestershire Sauce are gluten free.  Read the ingredients to make sure nothing has changed.

<u>**Cookies & Energy Bars**</u>: There are quite a few good tasting gluten-free cookies on the market:
- Glutino's Chocolate Chip cookies, about 60 Calories each
- Glutino's Chocolate Vanilla Creme cookies, about 60 Calories each
- Glutino's Vanilla Creme cookies, about 65 Calories each
- Kinnikinnick's Ginger Snap cookies, about 40 Calories each
- Udi's Chocolate Chip cookies, about 95 Calories each
- Udi's Ginger cookies, about 90 Calories each
- Udi's Oatmeal Raisin cookies, about 90 Calories each
- Udi's Snicker Doodle cookies, about 90 Calories each

**Energy Bars:**  An energy bar is a convenient and sometimes healthy snack. But be careful to choose a brand that comes with protein, vitamins, and minerals, rather than high fructose, corn syrup or sugar. The following are five gluten-free energy bar manufacturers. (There are others.)
- Bumble Bar Organic Energy Bar (about 200 Calories per bar)
- Macrobars Organic Peanut Protein (about 260 Calories)
- NuGo 10 Raw Natural Energy Bar (200 Calories)
- Pure Organic Raw Fruit & Nut Bar (about 200 Calories)
- Raw Revolution Organic Food Bar (about 200 Calories).

<u>**Frozen Entrees**</u>: Most larger supermarkets have a reasonably good selection of frozen entrees.  At this writing, Amy's and Artisan Bistro sell more gluten-free frozen entrees than any other manufacturer.  Smart Ones makes two gluten-free entrees.  Glutino offers two gluten-free frozen entrees, although each contain 400 Calories, and are not included in the following list.

- Amy's Quinoa, Black Beans, Butternut Squash & Chard (**240 Cal**)
- Amy's Black Bean & Cheese Enchilada (**240 Cal**)
- Amy's Mushroom Risotto Bowl (**240 Cal**)
- Amy's Sweet & Sour Asian Noodle Bowl (**250 Cal**)
- Amy's Vegetable Parmesan Bowl (**260 Cal**)
- Amy's Brown Rice & Veggies Bowl – Light in Sodium (**260 Cal**)
- Amy's Brown Rice, Black-eyed Peas & Veggies Bowl (**290 Cal**)
- Amy's Teriyaki Bowl (**290 Cal**)
- Amy's Asian Noodle Stir Fry (**300 Cal**)
- Amy's Vegetable Lasagna (**300 Cal**)
- Amy's Thai Stir-Fry (**310 Cal**)
- Amy's Tofu Scramble (**320 Cal**)

- Artisan Bistro Wild Alaskan Salmon (**200 Cal**)

- Artisan Bistro Chicken Parmesan Bake (**200 Cal**)
- Artisan Bistro Turkey Cheddar Bake (**240 Cal**)
- Artisan Bistro Wild Alaskan Salmon Bake (**240 Cal**)
- Artisan Bistro Thai Style Yellow Curry with Chicken (**240 Cal**)
- Artisan Bistro Cheddar Beef Bake (**250 Cal**)
- Artisan Bistro Sesame Ginger with Salmon (**270 Cal**)
- Artisan Bistro Coconut Lemongrass with Chicken (**270 Cal**)
- Artisan Bistro Spiced Chicken Morocco (**270 Cal**)
- Artisan Bistro Albacore Tuna Bake (**280 Cal**)
- Artisan Bistro Thai Style Red Curry with Beef (**280 Cal**)
- Artisan Bistro Chicken Citron (**280 Cal**)
- Artisan Bistro Wild Alaskan Salmon with Pesto (**310 Cal**)
- Artisan Bistro Savory Turkey (**330 Cal**)
- Artisan Bistro Southwest Style Beef (**330 Cal**)
- Artisan Bistro Ginger Chicken (**350 Cal**)
- Artisan Bistro Beef with Mushroom Sauce (**350 Cal**)
- Artisan Bistro Wild Alaskan Salmon Cake (**370 Cal**)

- Smart Ones Lemon Herb Chicken Piccata (**250 Cal**)
- Smart Ones Santa Fe Style Rice & Beans (**290 Cal**)

**<u>Fruits and Vegetables</u>**:  Fresh fruits, berries, greens and vegetables are naturally gluten free and generally safe. Most canned fruits and vegetables are gluten-free, but some are not.  Single-ingredient frozen fruits and vegetables are generally gluten free, but frozen fruits and vegetables with multiple ingredients frequently contain gluten.  Generally, more ingredients in a food increase the chance for trace gluten.  Read labels carefully or contact the manufacturer to determine if a particular product is processed in a factory or on manufacturing lines shared with gluten-containing products.

**<u>Legumes and Rice</u>**:  Legumes (lentils, beans, etc) are naturally gluten free, but there is always the risk of cross-contamination during processing and handling.  And be wary of canned lentils, beans, etc that have added ingredients.  "If in doubt, go without."

Brown Rice, white rice, long-grained rice, sticky rice and wild rice are all naturally gluten-free.

**<u>Meat, Poultry & Fish</u>**: Fresh meat, poultry and fish generally are safe on a gluten-free diet if they are not gluten cross-contaminated at a supermarket or butcher shop.  (Realize that the display cases in many stores contain fans that circulate air that could cross-contaminate unprotected meat, poultry and fish.  When in doubt choose meat, poultry and fish covered in plastic wrap.)

On the other hand, packaged processed meats, such as hams, bacon, sausages and luncheon meats, could contain gluten.  Look for packaged processed meat products labeled gluten-free.  Beware of meats and poultry with added ingredients that make them  ready-to-cook meals.  Most are not safe on a gluten-free diet because the store might have used unsafe ingredients when repackaging the food.  Avoid these products.

There are plenty of gluten-free **deli meats**. All of Boar's Head's products are gluten-free and Hormel and Hillshire Farms both make packaged gluten-free meats. But be wary of cross-contamination by shared slicing machines at the deli counter. To make sure deli meat or cheese are gluten free, choose pre-packaged products.

There are lots of **hams** that are considered gluten-free to 20 ppm, although most are not labeled gluten-free. Again check with the manufacturer.

GF **bacon** is widely available. A partial list includes:  Applegate Farms, Boar's Head, Jones Dairy Farm, and Wellshire Farms.  The following is a partial list of low-calorie gluten-free bacon: Jones Turkey Bacon (35 Calories per slice) and Wellshire Farms Turkey Bacon (40 Calories per slice).

Many **hot dogs** are gluten-free, and a few are labeled gluten-free.  A partial list follows: Jennie-O Turkey Franks (95 Calories each), Applegate Chicken Hot Dog (60 Calories each) and Turkey Hot Dog (50 Calories each).

The following is a partial listing of GF **burger patties**: Jennie-O Turkey Burgers (200 Calories each), Applegate Turkey Burgers (140 Calories each) and Beef Burgers (195 Calories each).

GF **veggie burgers** are produced by Amy's, Dr Praeger's and others: Amy's Bistro Veggie Burger (110 Calories) and Sonoma Veggie Burger (140 Calories) and Dr. Praeger's California Veggie Burger (110 Calories).

Many **sausages** contain bread crumbs as a filler, so check labels carefully before buying. In addition, even if the sausage does not include a gluten ingredient, it may have been manufactured on equipment that also processes gluten-containing sausage. The following is a partial list of GF sausage manufacturers: Al Fresco, Applegate Farms, Jones Dairy Farm, Smithfield and Wellshire Farms.  (We just tested an Al Fresco chicken sausage, and found it to be tasty, low calorie and gluten-free.  Al Fresco sausages are sold in many supermarkets.)

Canned **tuna and salmon** produced by Chicken of the Sea and by Bubble Bee are gluten free.

**<u>Milk and Dairy Products</u>**: Most milk and many dairy-based products are gluten-free.

Plain, unflavored milk, butter, plain yogurt, fresh eggs and many cheeses are gluten-free. Some ice creams are gluten-free.  And many flavored yogurts are gluten-free. Check the ingredients to be sure.

**Milk Substitutes:**  Soy, rice and almond milk are most often gluten-free, but some are not.  Check the labels.  (Soy, rice and almond milk may be substituted for cow's skim milk provided the calorie count is close.)

**Yogurt**:  All varieties of Chobani and Yoplait yogurt, including flavored varieties, are gluten free.  Yoplait Light in the 6 oz container has 90 Calories.

**Cheeses**: Most cheeses are naturally gluten-free.  One slice (1 oz) of light cheese has about 70 Calories. Beware of cheese that has been sliced and repackaged at a supermarket.  It might be cross contaminated.  Usually, it is safer to buy cheese that has been packaged at the manufacturer's plant.

**Cottage Cheese**: Breakstone, Cabot, Humboldt and others make fat free, gluten-free cottage cheese.

**Ice Cream**: Although many ice cream products are gluten free, some are not. Also consider GF frozen fruit pops. All of Skinny Cow's ice cream bars are gluten free: Chocolate Truffle Bar (100 Calories), Caramel Truffle Bar (100 Calories) and Fudge Bars (110 Calories).

**Oils, Nuts & Popcorn:**  Most oils (olive, canola, etc), nuts, and popcorn varieties are gluten free.  Nuts are naturally gluten free.  But beware of nuts and popcorn with added flavorings that might contain gluten.  Some popcorn brands that are considered gluten free are Jolly Time, Newman's Own and Orville Redenbacher's.

**Peanut Butter**: Arrowhead Mills and Smart Balance peanut butter are gluten free (about 95 Calories per tablespoon.)

**Mayonnaise**:  At this writing, Hellmann's and Best Foods regular and light mayonnaise are gluten free. (light is 35 Calories per serving)

**Non-Stick Cooking Spray**: Original Pam, Mazola and Wegman's store brand cooking sprays are gluten free.

**Pasta**: Fortunately, there are a number of gluten-free pastas available, in different shapes and sizes.  Choose gluten-free pasta made from rice or corn rather than wheat. Surprisingly, many of these gluten-free varieties are quite good, making it possible to serve gluten-free pasta whose taste is very close to wheat-based pasta.  The following manufacturers make gluten-free pasta: Ancient Harvest, Andean Dream, Bionaturae, Jovial, DeBoles, DeLallo, Le Veneziane, Lundberg, Riso Bello, Rizopia, Ronzoni, Rustichella D'Abruzzo, Sam Mills and Tinkyada.

**Salad Dressings**: When buying vinaigrette-type salad dressings look for cider or balsamic vinegar, not distilled vinegar on the food label. (Distilled

vinegar is made from gluten grains.)  The following salad dressings are gluten free:
- Annie's Lite Raspberry Vinaigrette (20 Calories per tablespoon)
- Annie's Lite Italian Dressing (23 Calories per tablespoon)
- Annie's Lite Honey Mustard Vinaigrette (20 Calories per tablespoon)
- Annie's Lite Herb Balsamic Vinaigrette (25 Calories per tablespoon)
- Annie's Lite Gingerly Vinaigrette (20 Calories per tablespoon).
- Gazebo Room Lite Greek Salad Dressing (20 Calories per tablespoon)
- Ken's Lite Options Italian w/ Romano & Red Pepper (23 Cal per Tbsp)
- Newman's Own Lite Balsamic Vinaigrette (13 Calorie per tablespoon)
- Newman's Own Lite Roasted Garlic Balsamic (25 Calories per tablespoon)
- Newman's Own Lite Red Wine Vinaigrette & Olive Oil (25 Cal per Tbsp)
- Newman's Own Lite Low-Fat Sesame Ginger (18 Calories per tablespoon)
- San-J's Tamari Sesame Salad Dressing (20 Calories per tablespoon)
- San-J's Tamari Ginger Salad Dressing (13 Calories per tablespoon)
- Sophia's Oil-Free Cilantro & Lime (5 Calories per tablespoon)

**Soups** (See Appendix C page 132 for a list of GF soup.)
Amy's Kitchen: A great many of Amy's 29 soups are considered gluten-free to 20 ppm.
Bookbinders Specialties: This gourmet soup company has 11 gluten-free soups. All are tested to below 20 ppm, and are available by mail order or in U.S. supermarkets in the northeast.
Frontier Soup: Frontier makes 28 varieties of gluten-free soup mixes. All are certified to below 5ppm of gluten. Frontier Soup mixes are available online and at upscale supermarket chains.
Imagine Foods: Imagine Foods claims all varieties of its soups are gluten-free to 20 ppm except for Organic Creamy Chicken and Imagine Bistro Bisques. Imagine soups are usually found in the "natural foods" section of supermarkets.
Pacific Foods: Almost all Pacific's soups are gluten free. Most often Pacific soups are found in the natural or health food section of a supermarket, although in some stores they are next to conventional soups.
Progresso: Choose from Progresso's many gluten-fee varieties tested to 20 ppm.

**Stock, Broth & Bouillon**: Stock is made by simmering vegetables, bones, meat scraps, etc, and is the best base for soups, stews, and sauces. Unfortunately stock is rarely found on supermarket shelves.  Broth is stock with added salt and can be used in the same way as homemade stock --

although broth is not as rich and complex as stock.  Bouillon is dehydrated stock formed into cubes or granules.  It is convenient but is typically processed with large amounts of sodium and other additives.  Thus the liquid it produces is almost flavorless.

Kitchen Basics makes gluten free Chicken, Beef, Vegetable, Turkey, Seafood, Veal, Unsalted Chicken and Unsalted Beef stock.  Pacific Foods sells gluten free vegetable broth, mushroom broth, beef broth and chicken and vegetable stock.  College Inn's garden-vegetable broth, organic-beef broth, tender-beef bold stock and white wine & herb broth are all considered gluten-free to 20ppm.  Hormel's vegetable, beef and chicken bouillon cubes are gluten free.

## Miscellaneous

We put food products in this category that did not seem to fit anywhere else.
Pancake Syrup: Hungry Jack Lite Syrup (25 Calories per tablespoon ), Log Cabin Lite Syrup (25 Calories per tablespoon) and Vermont Maid Lite Syrup (30 Calories per tablespoon) are gluten free.

# Appendix C
# Gluten-Free Soup*

| Soup Description | Calories* |
|---|---|
| Amy's Vegetable Barley Soup | 70 |
| Progresso Chicken Rice with Vegetables Soup | 80 |
| Amy's Alphabet Soup | 80 |
| Pacific Chicken Noodle Soup | 90 |
| Progresso Vegetable Classics Garden Vegetable Soup | 90 |
| Amy's Split Pea Soup | 100 |
| Pacific Butternut Squash Bisque | 110 |
| Amy's Cream of Tomato Soup | 110 |
| Progresso Traditional Manhattan Clam Chowder | 110 |
| Pacific Roasted Red Pepper & Tomato Soup | 110 |
| Amy's Mushroom Bisque with Porcini | 120 |
| Amy's Pasta & 3 Bean Soup | 130 |
| Pacific Chicken Spinach Penne Soup | 140 |
| Amy's Hearty Minestrone with Vegetables Soup | 150 |
| Amy's Summer Corn & Vegetable Soup | 150 |
| Progresso Vegetable Classics Lentil Soup | 160 |
| Amy's Tuscan Bean & Rice Soup | 160 |
| Progresso Hearty New England Clam Chowder | 180 |
| Progresso Potato Broccoli & Cheese Chowder | 200 |

* Calories per serving. When the Daily Meal Plan menu specifies soup, have only one serving (8 ounces) unless stated otherwise. (Note cans of soup usually contain about two servings.) See page 121 for additional gluten-free soup manufacturers.

# Appendix D
# Frozen Food Safety

Increasingly, food giants like ConAgra, Nestlé and others that supply Americans with processed foods concede that they cannot ensure the safety of their food products. Frozen foods can pose a particularly serious safety problem because unsuspecting consumers buy frozen foods for their convenience and incorrectly believe that cooking frozen foods is a matter of taste – not safety.

Still the food industry says that extensive outbreaks of food-borne illness are rare, even though it is well-known that most of the millions of cases of food-borne illness every year go unreported or are not traced to the source. For example, each year approximately 40,000 cases of salmonella poisoning are reported in the United States – but perhaps as many as one million cases go unreported. (Salmonella is a type of bacteria most often found in poultry, eggs, unprocessed milk, meat and water.) Recently salmonella pathogens in some frozen meals have sickened thousands of people.

How could this happen? First, the supply chain for ingredients in processed foods – from flour to fruits and vegetables to flavorings – is becoming more complex and global in the drive to keep food costs down. As a result, government and industry officials concede that almost every food ingredient is now a potential carrier of pathogens. A further complication is that a large number of food companies subcontract processing work to save money and don't require suppliers to test for pathogens. In fact, companies often don't even know who is supplying their ingredients.

In addition, many frozen-food manufacturers have stopped cooking their products at high temperatures, a tactic they call the "kill step," which is intended to eliminate any lingering microbes. Frequently this process step turns some of the frozen food ingredients into mush. So, instead the "kill step" has been shifted to consumers. For example, ConAgra has added food safety instructions to its frozen meals, including the Healthy Choice brand. A typical "frozen-food safety" instruction offers this guidance: "Internal temperature needs to reach 165°F (74°C) as measured by a food thermometer in several spots."

Moreover, General Mills, now advises consumers to avoid microwaves altogether and cook their frozen pizzas only in a conventional oven.

**<u>Bottom line</u>**: To be safe, always cook frozen foods so that the internal temperature reaches 165°F (74°C) as measured by a good food thermometer.

# Appendix E
# Exercise Smart

Our bodies are just not built to be immobile and passive. The sad fact, however, is that after years of education and information programs by government agencies, medical associations   and  insurance companies, relatively few  Americans  engage in  regular
planned exercise – despite the reality that we need to be active to keep our systems working efficiently and rid ourselves of emotional tension. Moreover, exercise burns calories, speeds up your metabolism and is an invaluable part of any weight control program.  There are two ways to become more physically active: 1) Increase the physical activity in your daily life; and 2) Start on a regular exercise program.  Better still would be a combination of both. Simply stated there are three basic types of exercise: aerobic, stretching and strengthening.

**Aerobic Exercises** (also called "cardio") condition your cardiovascular system. Aerobic exercises, such as jogging, swimming, cycling, brisk walking, skipping rope, and many others, are typically deep breathing and continuous, with rhythmic and repetitive contractions of your large muscle groups. The trait most aerobic exercises have in common is that they make you work hard and require you process a great deal of oxygen.

Some typical aerobic exercises are:  Most strenuous include bicycling, cross-country skiing, dancing (aerobic), hiking in rugged terrain, ice hockey, jogging, jogging in place, rowing, skipping rope, stair climbing, and stationary cycling.  Somewhat less strenuous are basketball, field hockey, calisthenics, handball, racquetball, skiing (downhill), soccer, squash, tennis (singles), volleyball, and walking (briskly). Least strenuous aerobic exercises consist of badminton, baseball, bowling, croquet, dancing, gardening, golf (carrying or pulling clubs), horseback riding, housework, ping-pong, shuffleboard, softball, tennis (doubles) and walking (moderate to leisurely).

**Stretching-type Exercises** such as yoga, tai chi, Pilates and to a lesser extent calisthenics can improve your flexibility – and some of the exercises can make you somewhat stronger.

As you age you inevitably start to loose flexibility. Your gait becomes stiffer; you can't stand quite as upright as you used to; it becomes tougher to bend over; and you have difficulty turning your neck. Regardless of your age, however, stretching can make you more flexible, less injury prone, and can reduce the pain and discomfort associated with tight muscles and shortened tendons. Realize, however, that stretching exercises do not condition your heart and lungs. Stretching exercises are fine as long as they are performed in addition to rather than in place of an aerobic exercise.

Most experts do recommend stretching before and after an aerobic or strength routine. However, never stretch cold muscles and always do some form of warm up prior to stretching.  Stretch slowly and hold gently. You should stretch to the point of feeling a mild pull, but you should never feel pain.  And when you stretch – do not bounce.

**Muscle Building and Strengthening** Exercises, e.g., weight lifting, use of the machines found in fitness centers and isometrics.

Once more, as you age you loose muscle mass, your bone density decreases and you lose strength. Exercises like weight lifting strengthen your muscles, bones and joints. Strengthening exercises also reduce your risk of developing osteoporosis, a severe bone-loss disease, which can lead to easily fractured bones and all the complications that often follow. Strong muscles not only allow you to lift a sleepy four-year old out of a car without difficulty and lug groceries up to a second floor apartment, but as with increased flexibility, strong muscles also make you less injury prone. Moreover, because **muscle uses many more calories than fat, when you replace fat with muscle, your metabolism actually speeds up.**

For everything you need to know about exercise see *Exercises Smart - U.S. Edition,* an eBook by Earl Simmons also published by NoPaperPress.

# NoPaperPress eBooks and Paperbacks

100-Day Super Diet-1200 Cal*  
100-Day Super Diet-1500 Cal*  
100-Day No-Cooking Diet-1200 Cal*  
100-Day No-Cooking Diet-1500 Cal*  
90-Day Smart Diet-1200 Cal*  
90-Day Smart Diet-1500 Cal*  
90-Day No-Cooking Diet - 1200 Cal*  
90-Day No-Cooking Diet - 1500 Cal*  
90-Day Perfect Diet - 1200 Cal*  
90-Day Perfect Diet - 1500 Cal*  
60-Day Perfect Diet-1200 Cal*  
60-Day Perfect Diet-1500 Cal*  
50-Day Flex Diet-1200 Cal*  
50-Day Flex Diet-1500 Cal*  
30-Day Quick Diet - Women*  
30-Day Quick Diet for Men*  
30-Day No-Cooking Diet*  
30-Day Diet - Women - Metric*  
30-Day Diet for Men - Metric*  
25 Day Easy Diet-1200 Cal*  
25 Day Easy Diet-1500 Cal*  
25-Day No-Cooking Diet  
10-Day Express Diet  
10-Day No-Cooking Diet*  
7-Day Diet for Women*  
7-Day Diet for Men*  
7-Day No-Cooking Diets*  
90-Day Gluten-Free Diet-1200 Cal*  
90-Day Gluten-Free Diet-1500 Cal*  
30-Day Gluten-Free Quick Diet*  
30-Day Gluten-Free No-Cooking Diet*  
7-Day Diet for Women - Metric*  
7-Day Diet for Men - Metric  
7-Day Gluten-Free Express Diet*  
7-Day Gluten-Free No-Cooking Diet*  
90-Day Vegetarian Diet-1200 Cal*  
90-Day Vegetarian Diet-1500 Cal*  
30-Day Vegetarian Diet*  
7-Day Vegetarian Diet*  
Weight Loss for Women*  
Weight Loss for Women - Metric  
Weight Loss for Women - UK  
Weight Loss for Men*  
Maximum Weight Loss - 1200 Cal*  
Maximum Weight Loss - 1500 Cal*  

Weight Loss for Men - Metric*  
Maximum Weight Loss- 1200 Cal*  
Maximum Weight Loss- 1500 Cal*  
Weight Control - U.S. Edition*  
Weight Control - Metric. Edition  
Prof Weight Control Women - U.S.  
Prof Weight Control Women - Metric  
Prof Weight Control Men - U.S.  
Prof Weight Control Men - Metric  
Weight Maintenance - U.S. Ed*  
Weight Maintenance - Metric. Ed*  
Weight Maintenance - UK Ed  
Weight Loss for Senior Men*  
Weight Loss for Senior Women*  
Eat Smart - U.S. Edition*  
Eat Smart - Metric Edition  
30-Day Mediterranean Diet  
Exercise Smart - U.S. Edition*  
Exercise Smart - Metric Edition  
Exercise Smart - UK Edition*  
Total Fitness - U.S. Edition  
Total Fitness - Metric Edition  
Total Fitness - UK Edition  
Total Fitness for Women-U.S. Ed*  
Total Fitness for Women - Metric  
Total Fitness for Women - UK Ed  
Total Fitness for Men - U.S. Ed*  
Total Fitness for Men- Metric Ed*  
Total Fitness for Men - UK Ed  
Senior Fitness - U.S. Edition*  
Senior Fitness - Metric Edition*  
Senior Fitness - UK Edition*  
Computer Diet - U.S. Edition*  
Computer Diet - Metric Ed*  
Reliable Weight Loss - U.S. Ed  
101 Weight Loss Tips*  
101 Healthy Eating Tips*  
101 Lifelong Fitness Tips*  
101 Weight Maintenance Tips  
101 Weight Loss Recipes  
101 GF Weight Loss Recipes  
101 Veggie Weight Loss Recipes*  
30-Day Mediterranean Diet*  
90-Day Mediterranean Diet - 1200 Cal*  
90-Day Mediterranean Diet - 1500 Cal*  

* These titles are available as both ebooks and paperbacks. Our ebooks are sold by Amazon, Apple, Google, Barnes & Noble and Kobo, but our paperbacks are only sold by Amazon.

# Disclaimer

This book offers general meal planning, nutrition and weight control information. It is not a medical manual and the authors do not claim to be medically qualified. Everyone should have a medical checkup before beginning this gluten-free weight loss program. Moreover, the physician conducting the medical exam should be made aware of and should approve this diet. Because commercial food ingredients and formulations can change at any time, adults with celiac disease or gluten sensitivity should be particularly careful and double check the ingredients in the foods listed in this book to be sure they are gluten free. We recommend that you do not solely rely on the information presented here and that you always read labels, warnings, and directions before using or consuming a product. For additional information about a product, please contact the manufacturer. The content on this site is for reference purposes and is not intended to substitute for advice given by a physician, pharmacist, or other licensed health-care professional. You should not use this information as self-diagnosis or for treating a health problem or disease. Contact your health-care provider immediately if you suspect that you have a medical problem. Additionally, while the authors and publisher have made every effort to ensure the accuracy of the information in this book, they make no representations or warranties regarding its accuracy or completeness. Further, neither the authors nor publisher assume liability for any medical problems that might result from applying the methods in this book, or for any loss of profit, or any other commercial damages, including but not limited to special, incidental, consequential or other damages, and any such liability is hereby expressly disclaimed.